DOCTOR'S NOTES

More Incredible True Tales from a GP's Surgery

Dr Rosemary Leonard

with David Meikle

headline

First published in 2014
by HEADLINE PUBLISHING GROUP

1

Cataloguing in Publication Data is available from the British Library

ISBN 978 0 7553 6208 0

Typeset in Baskerville by Avon DataSet Ltd,
Bidford-on-Avon, Warwickshire

Printed and bound by CPI Group (UK) Ltd, Croydon, CR0 4YY

HEADLINE PUBLISHING GROUP
An Hachette UK Company
338 Euston Road
London NW1 3BH

www.headline.co.uk
www.hachette.co.uk
www.drrosemaryleonard.co.uk

AUTHOR'S NOTE

The essence of each of the stories in this book is based on my experience as a GP for twenty-five years. However, certain details have been altered and stories merged to protect the identities and confidentiality of patients and colleagues. The exceptions to this are Maggie and Sean who have given their permission for their stories to be used.

CONTENTS

CHAPTER ONE

THE DISAPPEARING PENIS

I tried to look at Joe's face but he was staring intently at his brown, Nubuck footwear. Perhaps, like me, he was trying to work out whether they were shoes or trainers. Whatever they were, they needed a good clean. I was certain, though, that he hadn't come to see me about a missing suede brush.

From the lack of eye contact and the way he was absent-mindedly picking around his fingernails and thumbs, I had an inkling what he was planning to talk to me about. He bowed his head, providing a complete view of his flaky scalp. I was fairly certain that neither the flakes nor the bald patches were the reason for his appointment.

Joe's gaze lifted slightly from the grubby shoes, up his

beige chino trousers towards his groin, then down again. 'It's disappeared,' he informed me in an embarrassed whisper.

'What's disappeared, Joe?' I asked gently.

'I, em . . . it's . . . well, you know . . . it's just disappeared. What am I going to do, doctor?'

Joe had developed a mixture of accents over the course of his life, sounding mainly from London but with a variety of different twangs thrown in. His father had been in the army and had taken Joe with him all over the world. He spoke well, to be fair, but added an irritating 'you know' to some of his sentences. I heard a footballer once who said 'you know' in every sentence; Joe wasn't that bad, but I wished he would ease up on the phrase.

'I'm here to help, Joe,' I reassured my miserable patient. 'That's why I'm sitting in this chair, ready to sort things out. It's my job. This is all in confidence, so you can tell me whatever you like.'

The frown on Joe's weather-beaten face eased a little, although he was still cautious. 'But you'll be taking notes, won't you?'

'Consultations between a doctor and patient are completely confidential. None of this goes any further unless you give me permission to tell someone.'

'Reeeeaaaally?' Joe responded, spending several seconds eking out the word. The frown reappeared and his body stiffened up again.

'Yes, really,' I smiled.

The Disappearing Penis

'Ah, but what about your receptionists, then? They saw me coming in. Now, there's a loophole for you.'

'No loophole,' I answered, slowly and deliberately, to emphasise that there were, indeed, no loopholes.

'Yes, but it's no secret that I am here, you know. They saw me and I saw them,' Joe retorted, assuming the offensive position and trying hard to keep me on the back foot.

I batted straight back with the truth, 'Joe, they're not even allowed to tell anyone that you've been here! Aside from that, we have a superb team and they would never dream of uttering a word.' I stared straight back, not averting my gaze. I put my heart and soul into that look of reassurance because my patient came first.

My perseverance paid off. Joe nodded, stroked his chin, looked out of the window for a few seconds and turned his bloodshot eyes towards me. He managed a weak smile, nodded again, and relaxed in his chair.

'It's my penis, doctor, you know,' he muttered quietly. 'It's shrunk. It's gone down to nothing. There's absolutely nothing there any more. Telling you about this is the hardest thing I've done in my entire life. I took ages before deciding to come to see you.'

I was fairly sure his manhood hadn't deserted him overnight. 'When did this happen?'

'It's been getting smaller for some time . . .'

'What's some time? A couple of weeks? A couple of months?'

3

'Oh no, probably at least a couple of years now,' Joe admitted. 'But now it's gone altogether. I can't find it at all. Going to the toilet is a bit of a problem.'

I gestured with my hand, urging Joe to continue.

'Actually, going to the toilet is more than a problem – it's a serious issue,' Joe blurted out, his voice speeding up as he gave me the full facts. 'I can't hold my penis. I can't use a urinal, you know. I don't know which direction I'm going to pee in. I have to go and sit down in a cubicle. It's awful, doctor. It's awful.'

His brown eyes met mine again. They were moist and I wondered whether he was about to burst into tears. The great hulk of a man in front of me looked like a lost, little boy.

'Doctor, I can't have sex with my wife. I can't even let her see down there because it would be a disaster, you know.' Joe's next questions came all at once. 'Can you help me? Is there something you can do? Have you come across this before?'

'Yes, of course, this does happen. It's because—'

'Will I need an operation?' Joe butted in, becoming anxious again, with that frown forming rapidly as he spoke.

I was fairly sure I knew why his willy had disappeared and treating the underlying problem wasn't going to be easy. I'd known Joe for the last fifteen years and during that time I'd watched as his stomach expanded from just a small paunch above his trouser belt to a mountain of staggering proportions. Even now, I could see that the lower buttons of his shirt were fighting a losing battle, straining to cover the bulging skin underneath. I feared one of them might ping off at any moment and hit me in the eye.

'Joe, I need to examine you to see what's going on. Would you like a chaperone in here for the examination?'

My question caught Joe totally by surprise. 'A chaperone, Dr R? What on earth for? I've known you for years. Is this some stupid new rule dreamt up by 'elf 'n safety?'

That was more like the Joe I knew. I afforded myself a smile and a little laugh. 'No, it's just we have to be so careful now. I have to offer everyone a chaperone, when doing intimate examinations.'

'Well, I don't want one. You've never pounced on me before and I don't suppose you're going to now – especially with what I've just told you, you know, because I've only got a small, you know . . . it's only a tiny . . .'

'Yes, I know.'

The enormity of the situation, in Joe's mind, meant that he was becoming more and more stressed. He relaxed at times, when I gave an answer he wanted to hear, then went into panic mode as soon as he reminded himself about his lack of manhood.

I pulled the curtains around the couch while Joe undressed and checked back through his records. He'd never been a small man, but when I first met him he was only slightly overweight. Now he was very overweight. No, I thought again. He wasn't just overweight; that was being kind. Joe was obese.

As his girth increased, his blood pressure and sugar levels had soared upwards. His pancreas was now unable to produce enough of the hormone insulin, which normally controls sugar levels in the bloodstream and keeps them within the normal range. He was a Type 2 diabetic, taking medication.

I'd recorded the numerous conversations I'd had with him about the health merits of shrinking his waistline but it seemed the more I tried to give advice about eating a low-fat diet and drinking less booze, the more Joe indulged. He cheerfully admitted that taking an extra pill each day was an easier way to control his blood pressure than losing weight.

I recalled that he'd told me in the past: 'I like my food and so does the missus, you know. Barbara's a good cook. We only have one go at this life, Dr R. You've told me the risks, I know, but I'm going to enjoy myself.'

I steeled myself, took a deep breath, and slipped through the gap in between the curtains. Joe was lying on the couch. As instructed, he had undone his shirt and removed his trousers. I was greeted by the biggest stomach ever to reveal itself in the surgery. I could not remember ever seeing such a vast mound of flesh. Even in my days doing obstetrics, examining women carrying twins, I had never encountered such an enormous abdomen. An area of grey jersey was stretched around the lowest couple of inches, just covering his groin and the tops of his legs.

'May I take these down so that I can see what has happened?' I asked.

It was clearly a long time since there had been any functioning elastic in the top band of his underpants and they slipped down easily. Initially, standing by the side of the couch, I couldn't see any of his genital area at all. I had to move myself down towards his feet in order to get a view that wasn't obscured by his paunch. A few pubic hairs came into view, then I caught a glimpse of his scrotum. At first glance, there was no penis to be seen. But then, looking more closely at the top of his scrotum, I could just make out a small, pink, grape-like object with a hole in the middle. Found it!

'Joe, I just need to press a little bit on your lower tummy,' I explained, as I pushed hard on either side of the 'grape'. As I compressed the roll of fat at the bottom of his abdomen, more of his penis slowly appeared. I managed to find the whole of the glans penis, the area covered by his foreskin, and a couple of millimetres of the shaft. But that was all. The rest of what used to be Joe's pride and joy remained hidden from prying eyes, including mine.

'It hasn't disappeared,' I said. 'It's just been hidden by your, er, tum.'

'But my weight is around my middle and not down

there, surely? I can still feel my balls. Only just, mind you . . .'

'How much do you drink, Joe?' I ventured, realising that this might be a sore point.

'Eh? How much do I drink? What's that got to do with my old man vanishing? I don't drink that much, you know.'

'Well, your waistline is telling me that you drink a lot of booze, probably beer, although any alcohol is very fattening. I've known you long enough to tell you that, Joe. I believe you drink far too much.'

'Dr R, I can hold my drink. And I'm a big bloke, remember, so the quantity isn't much of an issue. I don't drink *that* much.'

However, I could tell that Joe drank a lot. I could detect last night's beer seeping through his pores as I examined him and I wasn't going to let this one go; his lifestyle would have to change. I gestured to Joe that I was finished and slipped back through the curtains towards my desk. He joined me, fully dressed, making huffing and puffing noises.

'Joe, when I have a stressful day, I admit to having a glass or two of wine. How much would you say that you drink in a day?'

Joe's ruddy complexion turned even ruddier as he sighed with exasperation and looked at me accusingly. 'I've always enjoyed a drink at lunchtimes and after work. So what, Dr R, so what?' He was sounding defensive.

The Disappearing Penis

Joe's jobs as a sales rep, nightclub bouncer and part-time barman had immersed him in a daily diet of fast food and copious amounts of alcohol.

'Joe, I have other patients to see,' I told him firmly. 'How much are you drinking every day?'

'Two pints at lunchtime.'

'And?'

'Six or seven pints in the evening . . . maybe eight or nine on a Friday or Saturday night.'

'Plus the two at lunchtime on weekends?'

'Yes,' he replied meekly, realising there was no way out now.

I was getting somewhere at last. 'Low strength, medium, or what?'

'I usually have pints of continental lagers . . . Some of the beer around here is too weak. It's like dishwater, you know.'

'Time for a lecture,' I said, checking online to make sure that my facts and figures were 100 per cent accurate.

'I didn't come here for a lecture,' Joe hissed.

I stood up, looked at my watch and gestured that he was allowed to leave, to put the entire matter back in Joe's court. I was keen to help him but I wasn't going to waste my time and his, and risk keeping other patients waiting, if he didn't want to be given assistance.

'OK,' he muttered, rolling his eyes to make sure I knew his feelings on the matter, 'go on, if you must.'

'Right,' I answered, trying not to sound too

triumphant. 'The "safe" limit for men – and who knows what is really safe – is between three and four units a day. The lager you are drinking is at least five per cent proof and so your "safe" limit is a pint or so.'

'A pint?' Joe laughed. 'Ha ha . . . Come on, Dr R. A pint? Wait until I tell the lads about this. All I can have on a night out is one pint? It won't touch the sides!'

I suppressed an inner chuckle as Joe scoffed at my suggestions. Beer wasn't the only thing that couldn't touch the sides.

'Yes, that's right,' I said. 'As you are drinking strong lager, that's your limit. If you drink a beer which is four per cent alcohol by volume, you can have a pint and a half.'

'This is getting ridiculous, you know,' Joe fumed, his ruddy face turning bright red. 'I'll be in the pub for about five minutes, then.'

'Look, Joe,' I warned. 'If you have seven pints of strong lager in an evening, you are using up your weekly allowance in one day. And, in a week, instead of having twenty-one units of alcohol, you are having 150 or more.'

'Eh?' Joe gasped.

'You are at risk from various cancers, hepatitis, cirrhosis of the liver, strokes, stomach disorders and a whole lot more. You already have Type 2 diabetes. Today I'm really worried about the size of your stomach.' The lecture continued. 'Now, you're on medication for your diabetes and I've suggested in the past that you should change your lifestyle. You need more than just pills to get you back on track.'

Joe gulped, stopped frowning and leaned across the desk. I had his full attention at last. 'Right, doctor.'

I laid it on thick. 'You have an enormous belly. Any alcohol is full of calories and you're taking in a lot more calories than you burn, just in beer. Those extra calories are being stored as fat, mainly in your belly. Add to that all the pizzas and fried foods that I know you enjoy – are you with me?'

'Yes, but I'm not enjoying this, you know,' Joe scowled. 'What about my diabetes?'

'You'll be surprised to learn that alcohol guidelines are the same for diabetics and non-diabetics. In your case, all of those carbohydrates from the beer make your blood sugars go up, then down again later.'

'Drop down again later?'

'Yes,' I continued. 'The body can't produce glucose, needed by the body when blood sugars are low. You see, the liver is busy dealing with the alcohol; in your case, an awful lot of alcohol.'

'Oh, I see,' Joe said, stroking his chin. 'So, taking everything into account, I should stop drinking.'

'It's not as easy as that,' I answered.

'Look, Dr R, I have very strong willpower and I can stop drinking now.'

'I'm not saying this would happen in your case,

but stopping drinking suddenly can have severe side effects. I've known people to have nausea, vomiting and hallucinations. It's a serious business. With such a dependency on alcohol, heavy drinkers can have seizures and the situation can be life-threatening.'

'Bloody hell,' Joe whispered. 'I'm done for.'

'No you're not,' I reassured him. 'There are various options open to you, but I want to try something straightforward first.'

'Straightforward?' Joe gasped. 'None of that sounds straightforward to me, you know. It sounds like I have only hours to live, my body is about to give up, and I'll never get my penis back!'

'I haven't forgotten about your penis,' I reminded him. 'This will all help to resolve your problem.'

'What do you want me to do?' Joe asked, looking puzzled.

'I want you to keep a diary.'

'A diary?' he moaned, looking totally opposed to the idea. 'What the hell would I want to keep a diary for?'

As Joe tapped the table, looking baffled by the diary request, there was a gentle knock on my door. Doreen, the senior receptionist, opened the door slightly and peered into the room.

'I'm really sorry to interrupt. There's a young lad in reception with a big bump on his head. I think the other doctors are carrying out examinations and the practice nurse has a bit of an emergency. Could you help me with this one?'

I waved a bunch of leaflets in front of Joe, left him to read them, and followed Doreen into reception.

In her mid-fifties and around five feet four inches tall, Doreen is our senior receptionist. She is a striking, well-built woman of Afro-Caribbean origin with an enormous bosom; I guess that she is an H Cup, but who would dare to ask? Inside, a big heart beats – and it has a cynical side. She is extremely good at sorting out those who are genuinely ill from those who think they are ill when they're not.

As we marched into reception, Doreen leading the way, I could tell she was concerned about this unexpected patient. She has an uncanny sixth sense about what to do in any situation and her instincts are usually on the right track.

'What's your name?' I asked as soon as I saw the boy sitting in the corner of the waiting room, holding his head.

'Ben.'

'What happened to you?'

'Well, I was playing football and the ball hit me on the head after a free kick. I was OK during the game but I'm feeling a bit dizzy now and I have a bad headache.'

'Ambulance,' I shouted over to Lizzy who had just come off the phone. 'Head injury.'

'It was only the ball,' Ben protested, pointing to his

head as if I needed my own head examined. 'The coach said I should pop in to see you, but I'll be fine.'

'Ben, haven't you been watching the news recently?'

'News about what?'

'Well, in extreme cases, heading a ball can lead to brain injuries. Football is coming under scrutiny at the moment.'

'Don't be ridiculous,' Ben laughed, standing up and revealing his height of well over six feet. He was tall for a lad of about fifteen, and I could see why he won most of the balls in the air.

'A football can travel at seventy miles an hour,' I informed him confidently, having read about football speeds on the BBC website.

I remembered a medical article which had reported that 'frequent headers' of a ball were shown to cause mild traumatic brain injuries. Scans revealed that five parts of the brain were damaged, affecting various processes such as memory and attention. I was fairly sure that Ben would be fine, but the lump on the back of his head needed checking out. I never take any chances with a head injury.

I could see that Ben had taken quite a blow and I was relieved when the ambulance arrived within ten minutes. It must have been a quiet day for them, as usually they take a lot longer for something that isn't life threatening. The crew came into the surgery with a stretcher and ensured that Ben's head was kept completely still while they moved him gently out of the surgery and into the ambulance.

Back to Joe, then. I hoped he had seen sense during his 'leaflet browsing' session.

'You said you wanted me to keep a diary,' he said as I arrived back in my room. 'Well, you know I'm a sales rep, so I need to keep everything logged anyway. I already jot down my whereabouts every day and make sure that my mileage is correct – what use is any of that to you?'

I could sense that he wasn't going to like my plan of action. 'We need to tackle your drinking. I can get you outside help – I can organise counselling – and I can sort out drugs to help with withdrawal but, in your case, I reckon that a lifestyle change is the answer. I want you to keep a diary to show how much you are drinking.'

'You what?' Joe bellowed, with a bright red face. 'Why would I want to keep a diary about my drinking?'

I had more suggestions up my sleeve. 'And I want you to have two alcohol-free days a week.' Having laid the foundations I felt confident enough to thrust a few more leaflets in front of the doubting Joe. They were NHS guides to sensible drinking, backing up everything I had said, including the two days on orange juice.

Joe could hardly argue with the evidence in front of him. The House of Commons Science and Technology Committee had checked out all the research. With time marching on, I decided enough was enough; Joe had had a plentiful supply of advice and literature. 'I've got to see the next patient now,' I said, getting to my feet. 'As I have explained to you, with the amount you are drinking, it could be dangerous to stop suddenly. I want you to read up on the effects of your massive intake, plus the benefits of cutting down and having two days of no drinking, and come back and see me in a month.'

'I'll give it a try,' Joe answered, clutching his information pack and staring at his enormous belly.

'Oh, and Joe, if you have any problems at all, come back at once. Remember that your body is used to a day packed with alcohol and it may grumble as you cut down.'

Patients came and went in a steady stream for the rest of the day. I was confronted with sniffles, coughs, man flu, woman flu, period pains and migraines. I was pleased to find solutions for all the ailments but I wanted to keep tabs on the football injury.

I buzzed through to reception. 'Doreen, did you hear any more about the lad who was hit by the football? I reckon he took quite a blow.'

'Not yet,' Doreen answered. 'I always worried about my kids playing ball games. I've been reading up about concussion and it says here to look out for dizziness and headaches. Ben had those symptoms, didn't he?'

'Yes, they'll carry out other tests at the hospital. He might have difficulty remembering things and he might be sensitive to light. I'm sure they'll tell him to have a break from football, whatever his symptoms. Would you mind checking to see what happened?'

I do have a need to follow everything through; at the end of the day, I like to know how my cases develop. It's not always as easy as it sounds, though – sometimes it takes weeks to get information from the various London hospitals which my patients attend. But if people come to me for treatment and advice, it really helps to know the whole story further down the line. It also prepares me for their next visits!

Doreen tapped on my door. 'Good news, I think. They say Ben has minor traumatic brain injury.'

'It is good news, really,' I explained. 'It sounds serious but it means there has only been minimum brain damage caused, and there aren't usually long-term complications. They'll tell him not to play for a while and monitor his progress. Any bleeding would have been a real cause for concern. I'm sure he'll be fine.'

The weeks passed and I heard no more about Ben. I was happy about that, and also pleased to hear no more from Joe – although, as the weeks went by, I began to wonder how he was doing. Had he actually taken any notice of the advice I'd given him?

If Joe was indeed 'self-detoxing', I knew he might have side effects such as nausea, fever or headaches and other symptoms. That was why I had told him to come back at any time. Some people can't adjust and are happy to continue in their old ways; others grab the opportunity for a new life. In some cases, a support system and more medical attention is required. It all depends on the individual.

Just over three months after Joe's examination, a familiar name appeared on my list of appointments. This was going to be interesting.

'Hello, Joe. How are you?'

I watched carefully as he strode into my consulting room. He had a fresh complexion, bright eyes, and a wide, wide smile.

'I'm not there yet,' he murmured cautiously. 'But what do you think?'

'You've lost weight, haven't you?'

The belly was still there, but there was certainly much less of it to be seen hanging over his trousers. The difference was astounding.

'I've lost twenty kilos,' the fit-looking Joe announced proudly.

'You didn't look confident when you left here a few months ago,' I reminded him. 'I was considering drugs to help you, with some extra support, too. How much are you drinking now?'

Joe beamed, glowing with that healthier complexion, and I could see that his blood pressure had dropped. He produced a small diary from his top pocket, opened it at the start and pointed to the page.

'Day one, I failed. I had six pints.'

'Oh,' I replied, trying not to sound too disappointed.

'Day two – seven pints.'

'I see,' I said, not convinced where the conversation was heading.

'Day three – five pints.'

'That's better,' I nodded. 'And was your diet improving? Not so many burgers and fries on your plate?'

'That's right,' Joe answered. 'At the end of the first week I was eating fresh vegetables, fish and fruit, as suggested in the leaflets. They said to avoid sugary food and drinks to help with my blood sugar, so I tried to get my head round that lot. On the fourth day I was down to four pints and for several days after that I was down to three.'

'That is still a lot. Bear in mind that you drink strong beer,' I reminded Joe, smiling and making sure that I didn't come across as too negative.

'I think this is the breakthrough. In the second week I got it down to two pints a day, but I was still drinking every day. In the third week I managed to avoid drinking on the Monday and Tuesday. That was hard. I went for long walks instead and drank loads of water. I found it hard to get to sleep and really enjoyed my two pints after the two alcohol-free days.'

'Well done!' I exclaimed. 'You are looking like a new man.'

'At the moment I am down to a pint and a half, and just managing to get through those two healthy, booze-free days. I don't know if I'm an alcoholic but I'm obviously dependent on it to some degree, you know.'

'You're not alone,' I told Joe. 'The NHS estimates that nine per cent of men and four per cent of women in the UK show signs of alcohol dependence. You'd built up a tolerance to alcohol. You had to drink more and more to achieve the same effect.'

'I have to tell you that I feel so much better now,' Joe beamed. 'I'm going to try to cut down even more and I'll stick to that healthy diet. I haven't felt like this in years. Oh, and something else is making a reappearance.'

'Yes, I was going to ask about that. Let's have a look.'

Joe eagerly slipped behind the curtain, keen to show me the size of his penis. His belly was indeed half its previous size and more of his manhood was showing.

'What do you think, Dr R? What do you think?'

'Well, Joe, there is an expression doctors sometimes use about weight gain in men. We say: "Gain an inch, lose an inch". For every inch of fat you put on around your middle, you lose an inch from your penis. It just gets buried in fat. And that is what happened to yours. It was still there – just buried.'

'Me and the missus are having sex again. It's not great, but it's getting better. Barbara says I have to lose another three stones.'

'Yes, that's another twenty kilos. You can do it.'

As Joe bounded out of the room and through reception, I felt a real sense of achievement. He was controlling his drinking, eating healthy food and getting plenty of exercise. Those had been my objectives when he first came to see me. I liked that phrase: 'gain an inch, lose an inch'. I decided I would have to use it again. I reflected on all the hundreds of obese patients there were here in South London and wondered how many inches they had lost in the 'crown jewels' area.

Joe had struggled to start with, but he looked and felt so much better after his change of lifestyle. Will it last? You know, I think he can do it.

CHAPTER TWO

STRANGE THINGS IN STRANGE PLACES

'My girlfriend has a sensitive problem.'

'What type of sensitive problem?' Lizzy the receptionist enquired, prepared for anything from a missed period to a mysterious rash and all sorts in between. She handled calls about sensitive problems all day, every day. That was her job and she performed it well.

My Rosendale surgery was busier than ever with the pre-Easter rush – and, as usual, time proved to be a formidable enemy. The telephones all seemed to be ringing at once. Any phones not ringing were merely enjoying a brief break, ready to explode into action without warning.

'There's something stuck up there and I can't get it

out,' the concerned male voice said in between intermittent buzzing sounds. 'She can't get it out either.
We're worried that it could be stuck in there for good.'

'I'm sorry, sir, it's a very bad line,' Lizzy said, raising
her voice slightly to cut through the crackle. 'Would you
mind repeating that? What's stuck – and where?'

The fading voice repeated the scant details once
more as Lizzy strained to hear. She persevered as the
poor line faded, then returned and disappeared again.
Lizzy has endless patience and a lovely nature. Patients
often say that she has a calming influence during that
crucial first point of contact. Sometimes she can be a
bit too soft and tries to get everyone fitted in, even
when there aren't the appointments available. I can cope
with that, except when I'm really tired, but it is far better
than having a receptionist who gives people a harsh
response.

Although this particular caller had chosen late
afternoon on Maundy Thursday to ring, the right person
was answering the call. Patience was vital here; we
didn't want someone in distress to be embarrassed and
disappear without medical help.

I had wandered into the reception area to collect the
pile of prescriptions waiting to be checked and signed,
and could see Lizzy's face twitching nervously. She also
had her hand over her mouth in an attempt to stifle any
suggestion of laughter. She was concentrating hard
on this unusual call and, as she glanced at me, I had a

feeling that this case would soon be heading in my direction. I heard her repeating the words 'sensitive problem'; not only was I the 'duty doctor', the one who took the majority of extra patients at the end of each surgery, but I was also the doctor with most experience in gynaecological problems.

I returned to my consulting room to sign the prescriptions. I continued writing while, in the reception area, the phones kept ringing and ringing and ringing. As soon as one call was completed, another took its place.

Although it had been the usual busy day before a bank holiday weekend, I had really enjoyed it. None of the patients had been rude or argued with me – that made a big difference to the way I felt by late afternoon. Many had been really friendly and asked what I was going to do over the long weekend.

I was interrupted from my writing by Lizzy knocking at my door. She strode in, looking puzzled. 'That call you overheard. It was a boyfriend and girlfriend, both jabbering away at the same time. The boyfriend would like you to call them back. It was difficult to make out exactly what the problem was because it was a bad line. All I could gather was that a foreign object is lodged in an unfortunate place.'

There were a couple of possible places, of course, but I think I established the location of the trouble spot. 'Is there anything else I should know?' I asked, spotting Lizzy's smirk.

'It was a bizarre call,' she explained. 'They were on a mobile and the signal wasn't very good so it was difficult to hear their exact words . . .'

'I'll call them back,' I told her, wondering what on earth the 'foreign object' was. 'I'm sure we'll get to the bottom of it, so to speak.'

Lizzy stood up and towered over me. She is an imposing figure, standing more than six feet tall with long, shining, black hair. She's Scottish and occasionally comes out with phrases from north of the border. When she goes shopping, she says she is 'going to get her messages'. I keep thinking about e-mails or texts, and can't get my head around going to the shops for messages.

I glanced up at Lizzy, whose friendly, deep-blue eyes flashed and reflected the bright, artificial lights in the surgery. The message I received from those shining eyes was: 'I've done all I can – now over to you.'

The broad Scottish accent confirmed her stance: 'Hopefully, on a better phone line you can get the rest of the details from the patient. The man was talking, with the woman chipping in to add occasional details, but I struggled to make much sense of it all. In the end, the woman said that they had to go and I didn't have a chance to get her name.'

On with the job then, I decided. The phone rang a few times and for a minute I thought there was going to be no reply. A male voice answered and I assumed that the boyfriend had taken the call. I concentrated hard, to make sure that my enquiry sounded tactful. 'Hello, it's Doctor Rosemary Leonard here. You wanted a call from the duty doctor?'

'Yes, thanks for getting back to me.'

'Who am I talking to?'

'My name is Kevin. My girlfriend's name is Gemma, but she's too upset to tell you what happened. She had a go at talking earlier, but she keeps breaking down. She's not injured. She's just crying and embarrassed.'

I decided to establish the facts straight away. 'I need to know exactly what happened. I'm here to help you. Just take me through it all from the start.'

Kevin began to provide his details in instalments and, after a minute or so, I knew about his supermarket security job and his relationship with Gemma, who worked on the checkouts. I decided to press for more intimate details – I couldn't spend all evening on the phone. I needed to know why he wanted medical advice.

'You told the receptionist that something was stuck.'

'That's right,' a sheepish-sounding Kevin whispered. 'It's gone right up inside her vagina.'

'Something? Could you tell me more?'

Every GP has encountered a patient with something inserted where it shouldn't have been placed, and we are all well practised at being supportive rather than shocked. But sometimes the situation is more than just embarrassing; foreign objects can cause serious problems, such as a ruptured anus or cervix, or torn vaginal walls. I really needed to find out exactly what was stuck inside the caller's girlfriend.

'It's an egg,' Kevin announced with more authority. He sounded as if he was starting to come to terms with the couple's predicament. 'It was an accident. We didn't want to call for help, but Gemma was getting worried.'

'What sort of egg? Was it one of those vibrating love eggs?'

'It's a . . .'

'Go on,' I pleaded, hoping for a breakthrough; I could see from my computer screen that other last-minute, pre-Easter calls were piling up. 'Please?'

'It's an Easter egg. It's a chocolate Easter egg.'

Now, I have come across carrots, cucumbers, celery, tomatoes, and all sorts of strange things in strange places. But, despite all of this and in all my medical experience, Gemma's chocolate intruder was a first.

'An Easter egg?' I spluttered. I decided the time was right to push for more information. I asked myself: was it a mini one, or family-sized? Did it still have the wrapping on? The conversation was all too much for Lizzy, who had stayed in the room after passing on the number to call; she dashed off back to reception, no doubt wondering if the egg was still in its presentation box.

'It's a Cadbury Creme Egg,' I was informed by Gemma's boyfriend, who sounded almost apologetic on the other end of the line. 'You know, one of those small ones they sell in packs of three for Easter. I bought a pack for Gemma and we had a bit of fun with one of the eggs.'

'Just the one egg then,' I said, trying my hardest not to giggle, but relieved we were not talking about a king-sized version.

'Yes, just the one egg. And it's lodged in there. It won't come out. No way. I've been poking around inside but I can't seem to reach it. Also, we can't really have proper sex with an Easter egg in there. Gemma doesn't want sex, anyway, until this is sorted out.'

I thought back over the events in my week. I had only just finished dealing with a newly married elderly patient who pleaded for performance-enhancing drugs; a widow enquiring about sex toys; and a gay patient who needed something to cool his ardour. Even with Easter approaching, I hadn't expected this type of seasonal treat.

I tried not to scold Kevin and remained matter-of-fact: 'What were you doing, putting an Easter egg in there? I have to say, I haven't come across this before.'

'Well, we normally use a love egg,' he explained, getting into his stride. 'It's a little vibrator, and we use it just before having sex. It makes Gemma very excited. They're great things. We bought a few online. It was a good offer.'

'Yes, but this is a chocolate one . . .' I replied, keen to nudge Kevin towards providing more details about the incident itself, and distancing myself from any information about their preference for vibrating sex toys.

'I operate the love egg by remote control – it works from a few metres away and you can remove the egg afterwards because there's a cord attached.' The conversation was getting ridiculous. 'I thought I would try something different,' Kevin continued, appearing to relish the memory of his recent exploits. 'I removed the real love egg and decided to try the Easter egg. I took the foil off, slipped it into her vagina, but forgot there was no cord to remove it. So it's lodged in there and won't come out.'

All in a day's work, I reassured myself.

'No foil, then,' I wrote down, hoping that the situation wouldn't deteriorate any further. Oh, how I regretted being on duty that Maundy Thursday evening. What was I getting myself into? Would the egg come out naturally? Would it melt?

'It was just for a laugh, really. I know I shouldn't have done it. Could you come to our house?'

I glanced at my surgery ceiling in disbelief. Was this really the reason the NHS was set up? Were GPs invented in order to go round to people's houses to remove Easter eggs from vaginas?

'Er . . . I can't come out for that. Home visits are for people who genuinely can't leave their homes. I can see you here, though – could you come to the surgery?'

'My mate's borrowed my car and Gemma says she

can't walk around with this egg inside her in case it starts melting. She says it will look as if she's messed herself.'

I suggested that, while white linen trousers would clearly not be a good idea, if she wore a skirt and put a sanitary pad in her pants she should be able to walk to the surgery. I could see from their address on the screen that they didn't live far away.

'Gems, could you walk round to the surgery? The doctor says she can't come to us.'

I heard a scream of 'no way' in the distance, which was then repeated down the phone by Kevin. 'She says she can't walk anywhere.'

'What about a taxi?'

'Too expensive, so we can't afford that,' Kevin replied, lobbing the Easter egg problem back into my court.

'OK, Kevin. To start with, Gemma should have a hot bath. She should sit in it for a while and sluice water around her vagina. She needs to rinse the chocolate out.'

'But then she'll get the chocolate and crème filling all over everywhere. Surely there must be some way of removing it intact?'

'It really doesn't matter if the egg melts and the filling goes everywhere. It will wash off. Please give it a try? After the bath, she should . . . she should . . . hello? Kevin?'

The line went dead. I tried to dial back, but there was no ringing tone. I assumed that Kevin's battery had died or the signal had faded completely again, so decided to plough on with my other work.

I spent the next couple of hours telling myself that there must have been a satisfactory outcome but I have to admit that Gemma's predicament did play on my mind while I dealt with the final patients of the day. I wondered what had happened.

Closing time approached; everyone at the surgery was ready to go home. We were all tired, as it had been such a busy day, but the Easter egg issue still remained unresolved. I decided to try to call them one last time. Gemma answered and I got straight to the point. 'Hello, it's Dr Leonard here again. I'm not sure what is going on with your phone – we were cut off earlier. I know all about your problem, though. Could you give me an update, please? Has the egg made an appearance?'

'Sorted, sorted,' I could hear Kevin proclaiming in the background. 'We've nailed it, we've nailed it.'

Help, I thought to myself. Surely they hadn't resorted to piercing the thing with nails to get it out?

'Well, I had a hot bath and all is well,' Gemma explained to my relief. 'I've never been so embarrassed. The bath changed colour to dark brown with white and yellow curdy bits, but I am so, so relieved. Apologies for the bad telephone line, but I managed to catch your advice about the hot bath.'

'Thank goodness,' I sighed. 'I think it's best to stick

to the right tools for the job in future . . . and, now that you can relax, may I wish you a happy Easter.'

I was pleased to hear there were no real health issues, everything was hygienic and there didn't seem to be evidence of any injury. A brown, chocolate-covered bath was a small price to pay for removal of the unwanted object and total peace of mind.

Just as I was leaving for the day, I bumped into my colleague, Dr Nazareen Khan, who was also hurrying home. Her parents are from Pakistan, but she is extremely English; the same can be said of her husband. If you hear either of their voices on the phone, you won't have a clue that their lineage is from the other side of the world.

'I've been put right off my Easter eggs this year, Naz. Do you celebrate Easter at home?' Naz was a Muslim, so this was something that had always intrigued me.

'I didn't used to, until we had the children. Before them we just celebrated Muslim festivals. But now the kids insist we celebrate Christmas and Easter, too. They soon sussed that Christmas means presents and Easter means chocolate. It's awful, really, that they should be so materialistic.' I listened intently as Naz described her family life. 'They are being brought up British, so they insist on being treated the same as their English friends. I did think of trying to make them give up something for Lent but my eldest, who is eight, promptly replied that I didn't starve myself during Ramadan, so that was a non-starter. They just want the best of everything!'

'Can't say I blame them! My two boys are just the same,' I laughed, as we locked up and set the surgery alarm.

A week later I took advantage of a few precious moments in my Friday lunch break, checking out my garden centre's online spring plant range. I'm a passionate gardener; apart from the thrill of growing flowers, fruit and vegetables, the hobby takes my mind off the plethora of problems during my day job. I was just reading about a thistle with 'erectum' in its name – possibly a cure for a disappearing penis – when the deafening phone shattered the silence and ended my daydream. Its shrill tone threatened me with another crisis.

'Dr Leonard, there's someone here to see you,' Doreen told me. 'He doesn't have an appointment.'

'Is it urgent?'

'I'll come through and explain,' Doreen suggested. We would be lost without her rapid grasp of situations and her knack of 'making the right call'. 'He won't go away,' she told me as she walked into my office, looking slightly concerned. 'He has a package with him.'

'A package? I hope it's not a bomb . . .'

The waiting room was beginning to fill up for afternoon surgery with pensioners coughing, children playing and pregnant women comparing notes. In the corner I could see a man, aged around thirty, with a tattoo of the devil on his forearm. He had rings in both ears, a footballer-style haircut, a small but noticeable beer belly, a T-shirt with a rather vulgar logo, and blue jeans with state-of-the-art holes in them. My unexpected visitor also had a couple of teeth missing at the front.

'Hello, I'm Kevin,' he grinned, which seemed to make the gap in his teeth look even wider.

I chuntered to myself as he bounded over in my direction; his belly wobbled like jelly and his jewellery jangled. I forced my gaze away from his partly toothed mouth. This had to be Kevin of Easter egg fame.

'How is Gemma?' I asked.

'She's good, really good,' he replied. 'I thought I'd come to thank you and bring you a present.'

'Oh, there's no need for that. We often deal with similar cases, although your situation was a bit different for obvious reasons. I'm glad everything turned out well in the end. Now, if you don't mind, I have to—'

'Here you are, doctor,' Kevin boomed for all to hear, revealing his present. 'You really helped us and I'm pleased to say that our sex life is back to normal. It's important to have a healthy sex life, don't you think?'

I smiled, recoiling slightly from hearing such a loud voice, and examined Kevin's present. It didn't look like a bomb. I tore off the wrapping to reveal . . . a large Easter egg. I thanked him and placed the package on the desk at reception and offered the treats to all comers. Much as I love chocolate, somehow the background to the case put me off having any myself.

Kevin said his farewells and I caught my first sight of Gemma standing beside their bright red, sporty-looking Ford Focus. She was leaning on the bonnet, with red sandals and a short black skirt, soaking up the warm spring sunshine. She had long, blonde hair, with a variety of streaks, and a plunging neckline which revealed a selection of tattoos.

Gemma looked in her mid-twenties and was obviously crazy about Kevin because she smothered him with hugs. I imagined more eggs would be on the agenda; I just hoped they weren't of the Easter variety.

I returned to my office and, later, as the last of the sun's rays bathed the surgery in an orange glow, my door vibrated slightly with three gentle taps. I recognised the spaces between the knocks; it was Dr David, keen for a catch-up at the end of the day.

'Come in,' I said at once. 'I know who has come knocking.'

I peered through the fading light to see his tall, slightly stooped figure inching towards my desk. The lateness of the hour had failed to ruffle his neatly parted, silvery hair, his tweed jacket remained perfectly buttoned, his red silk tie reflected those final darts of sunlight, his glasses were perched precariously on the end of his nose, and his bristling moustache, the exact colour of his hair, followed the line of this English gentleman's lips as he broke out into a smile.

Dr David has always looked the same to me. I've

known him for about twenty years and he is an exceptional product of Oxford. He walks, talks and breathes the place, and you can just tell that he is well-read, sharp as a tack and packed with knowledge.

Oxford has been a prestigious learning base for medicine since the fourteenth century. Lord Nuffield, famous as the founder of Morris Motors Ltd, helped to set up a clinical medical school in 1936. During the Second World War, medical students were sent there from London to escape the bombing and clinical student training really took off. Dr David wasn't studying then, I assume, but I believe he was a student at Oxford in the early sixties.

I trained in medicine at Newnham College, Cambridge. I was always fascinated by the college's history and can confirm that it is still 'for women only'. The college began life in a house for students in Regent Street, Cambridge, in 1871. In 1875, Newnham Hall opened and, before the First World War, its facilities included an impressive library and a laboratory. The building is set in acres of stunning gardens, which kept alive my avid interest in horticulture while I was there.

Later, I attended St Thomas' in London. That world-renowned medical school was founded in 1550, about five years after the sinking of the *Mary Rose* in Tudor times. St Thomas' Hospital itself dates back to the twelfth century, so I benefited from a wealth of tradition and learning. I always felt, though, that Dr David had profited from a more privileged upbringing, while I 'had to make my own way'.

'I've heard all about your . . . eggstraordinary experience,' Dr David joked, looking crestfallen as I winced and emitted a disapproving groan.

'Have you ever experienced anything like that?' I asked. 'I was happy that it all worked out in the end, but what a crazy phone call.'

'Well, I did have a patient with an electric toothbrush inside his back passage.'

'You what?' I gasped, glad to forget about the Easter egg and at the same time fascinated to hear this well-spoken English gent sharing his more unusual experiences.

'Right up there it was,' he continued, knowing he had my full attention.

'How did the toothbrush . . . er . . . get up there?'

'It was a form of sexual experiment, I believe. One chap held the toothbrush while the other chap received it, but the darned thing slipped out of sight.'

'You're having me on,' I laughed. 'You're making it up.'

'No, no, honestly – the fellow was so embarrassed to call me out. There was nothing I could do. It ended up as a hospital job.'

'Really?'

'Oh yes,' he exclaimed. 'The toothbrush was still working, you see. It was going round and round.'

'So did they wait until it stopped before trying to get it out?'

'Well, it wasn't quite as simple as that,' he answered evasively, dragging out the story in his own unique style.

'Go on,' I insisted.

'Well, they asked him about the battery and, unfortunately, he'd just put one of those long life ones in. The bloody toothbrush could have gone on forever. I understand that a delicate procedure was required to remove the object.'

'I can see that a hot bath wouldn't have worked in that case,' I responded as the beaming Dr David marched towards my door. He was obviously satisfied that his story had grabbed my attention without the need for any more of his awful puns.

'By the way, I do recall a couple of other incidents,' he informed me with a naughty smirk as he clutched the door handle.

'No, no, please. I can't take any more strange things in strange places.'

Dr David's story is a true account, I'm sure of that, and it prompted me to do some more research. I read that, over the years, some bizarre objects have been recovered from rectums. One prisoner, I am led to believe, had an entire toolbox in there. Not surprisingly, he died from bowel obstruction.

Doctor's Notes

Dr David's story also gave me a flashback to another incident that happened to me before I went into general practice. I was working at a sexual health clinic in West London – it was this training that was to prepare me for virtually any sexual problem as a GP. I tested visitors for chlamydia, gonorrhoea, HIV, syphilis, hepatitis, herpes, warts and thrush plus several other complaints. We had follow-up care, leaflets to hand out – in fact, I would say the clinic had everything covered. There are always shocks and surprises in store, of course. One incident in particular stayed with me.

It was a glorious summer's day, the sun streamed in through the clinic windows and I was feeling happy in my job. When a certain patient walked in, though, I should have smelled a rat.

In he came with a swagger – his bright, tight-fitting shirt and jeans hinted to me that he was gay. He was immaculately dressed with expensive shoes, not one blond hair out of place. One ear was pierced, a chain was round his neck, and he had a bracelet. I certainly welcomed gays, heterosexuals, transvestites and every other section of the population at the clinic – my only objective was to make sure that the individual was checked out and left my care with a clean bill of health.

'How may I help?' I asked as my new patient gingerly eased himself on to the chair opposite my desk. 'Shall we start with your name?'

'It's Peter,' he blurted out, keeping details to a minimum. He was a striking young man – about twenty-five, I would say – with a recent sun tan and muscles everywhere. They were bulging out of his bright yellow shirt and the garment was neatly tucked into his designer jeans.

'What can we do for you?' I asked.

'I would just like a health check,' he said, firmly, and I thought that was fair enough. Very sensible of him. 'I'm just back from the States.'

'You're gay?'

'Yes. I've had one or two adventures over there, so I thought I should get checked out.'

'Adventures? Well, this won't take long,' I assured Peter, gesturing towards the private room and an examination couch. I assumed that Peter had visited bathhouses in America. I'd read that these gay saunas or steam baths provided opportunities for sex. They were not brothels but traded as membership-only places where no money was exchanged.

The jeans came off and I took the usual swabs from his penis. These are called urethral swabs and test mainly for gonorrhoea and chlamydia. I inserted a thin cotton swab gently into the opening at the tip of his penis. I warned him that it might be uncomfortable and he winced slightly as I rotated it slowly and withdrew the sample. I carried on with my work and took a second swab.

'Well done,' I said encouragingly. I didn't want to deter him from coming back to the clinic again. 'Now, can I just check – you said you're gay – I presume that means I should check your back passage as well?' Not all gay men have sex via the anus, so I always ask first. Peter confirmed that I should check that area as well.

I asked him to lie on his side, facing the wall, with his legs bent so that his buttocks were at the edge of the couch. I reached for my proctoscope. This is a short, thin, plastic tube used to examine the inside of the rectum. The device is designed to look for abnormalities, such as warts, tears, sores, bleeding, discharge, polyps and changes in the anal lining.

In went the proctoscope and I thought – what on earth is that? At first all I saw was a brown lump and I thought it might be faeces. But it didn't look like any lump of faeces I'd ever seen before, because it seemed to be wriggling sideways. And then I saw two eyes. I looked again. Yes, there were definitely two small dark eyes inside his back passage. This was certainly a 'first' for me.

I felt like giving Peter a piece of my mind but managed to keep my composure. I was determined to remain totally professional and go exactly by the book. I decided to get some extra help. 'Would you mind waiting there for a moment?' I said, removing the proctoscope. 'I'll be back shortly. Please remain exactly as you are.'

I dashed off to find Gavin, the charge nurse. I knew

that he was gay and in a good position to help me address this bizarre situation.

'Gavin,' I gasped when I found him. 'You know those stories about gerbils? Well, I think I've got someone with one. I have a gay patient on my examination couch and I believe he has a rodent up there. I put in the proctoscope and could detect slight movement. Then I saw two eyes. Whatever this thing is, it has two eyes.'

Gavin was an easy-going, helpful nurse with a terrific sense of humour. He was well-read, had a vibrant personality and was someone you could rely on. 'Two eyes?' he quizzed me with a disbelieving look. 'Leave this to me.'

Gavin managed to remain calm and polite as he introduced himself to Peter. I passed the proctoscope in and we were both eyeballed directly by the visitor inside Peter's bowel. Gavin nodded at me, and then took the lead.

'What is up there? We can't go pulling it out until we know what it is.'

'It's a gerbil,' a meek, embarrassed voice responded. 'It's a very small gerbil.'

Gavin reminded Peter of the health risks. 'This is how you contract animal-borne diseases. The gerbil has been scratching your rectum. It's all raw and red in there. We need to get you sorted out.'

'I'm really sorry. I do realise. It just sort of . . . happened. I got carried away. I got in with the wrong crowd over in the States. It seemed a good idea at the time.'

'Not very kind to the gerbil, though,' Gavin commented.

We managed to remove the moribund gerbil and it was a horrible sight. Gavin disappeared out of the door with it. I was speechless – absolutely gobsmacked. I knew I shouldn't be judgemental about sexual practices between gay men; I had to stay objective. I was so pleased that I had left all the talking to Gavin.

I went off to carry out extra research in case I ever came across another rodent in a rectum. I read all about so-called 'gerbilling' or 'gerbil stuffing'. The article I studied said that live rodents were inserted for erotic pleasure. I went on to discover that objects found inside vaginas include part of a shoe tree, which had been in place for fifty-three years; a salt cellar; a large drinking glass; a fourteen-inch cucumber; a flashlight bulb; a pen and pencil set; a deodorant stick, which caused burns from the chemicals; and an aerosol can.

Sharp objects inserted where they shouldn't be can cause injury, leading to bleeding, and if left in place for more than a few hours can act as a focus for infection. This, in turn, can lead to a foul-smelling discharge. There could be pain, discomfort while passing urine, or pain in the pelvis. Even if you are using conventional sex toys, you must be sure to keep them clean. Sharing sex toys is risky – they must be washed between uses and it is advisable to put new condoms on them. If you don't, it is possible to spread infections. Cuts or sores, showing blood, will mean an increased risk of catching hepatitis B, hepatitis C and HIV.

A few days later, I was enjoying a day out at a shopping centre when I spotted Peter a mile off. He was strutting around in his usual attire at the bottom of the escalator. As the shoppers' treadmill I was on groaned and squeaked its way to ground level, I could see there was no escape. I bowed my head and attempted to sneak past. Doctors only deal with patients when on duty and don't want to pass the time of day in shopping centres discussing medical issues. That's my experience, anyway.

'I'm so sorry,' Peter told me as the final step of the escalator launched me on to the floor of the shopping centre. 'It won't happen again.'

'Hello there. I'm glad you're OK but I can't really discuss your case here. Make sure you go back to the clinic for a follow-up.'

'I've been back,' persistent Peter answered, cornering me in one of the shop doorways and making sure I heard what he had to say. 'You must have been on a day off. I saw Gavin himself. Everything is healing and I have the all-clear.'

'Good, I am pleased, but I really shouldn't be discussing this outside the clinic,' I reminded him.

'That's no problem,' Peter interrupted. 'I just wanted to say that Gavin has made me see the light. He's gay, yes?' I glanced around for an escape route. I couldn't go discussing the sexuality of the clinic staff with patients. 'I'll leave you alone. Just to say that Gavin really spelled out all the dangers and I am handing out "safe sex" leaflets to my circle of friends. I thought you should know. I owe it to you guys.'

'Good work,' I smiled, and melted into the crowds inside Marks and Spencer.

I looked forward to telling Gavin about Peter's rehabilitation. I imagined that the charge nurse would be taken completely by surprise.

'You'll never believe who is going around giving out "safe sex" leaflets all over London?' I exclaimed when I bumped into Gavin back at the clinic.

Gavin was delighted when I told him. 'If it means no more cases like that, let's give him a barrow load to hand out!'

Back in the Rosendale surgery, Dr David was still loitering at my door. 'Have a good weekend,' he bellowed, and I assumed that it was a general greeting for anyone within earshot.

On Sunday morning Dr David and I were due to work with SELDOC, or South East London Doctors on Call. This covers 25,000 patients in South East London. Usually, two doctors deal with the calls and another two or three colleagues are on the road carrying out home visits. I am a proactive supporter of SELDOC – it began life in 1998 when GP practices joined together to form an out-of-hours service. Doctors across Lewisham, Southwark and Lambeth agreed on a way to provide better care for patients. It provides urgent medical care for people in our part of the capital when GPs' surgeries are closed. Callers are asked for their name and address; the name of their doctor; details of the medical condition; and details of any medication being taken. The service operates for 365 days a year and I am immensely proud to play a role in the scheme.

I sorted out my desk, handbag and everything else while the persistent Dr David hovered at the door. He looked back at me and said, 'If I get any egg-related calls on Sunday, may I direct them to you, as you have such experience in these matters?'

'OUT!'

CHAPTER THREE

THE PERILS OF
FOREIGN MEDICINE

'Something has happened to my ears. Look at them. They are really ugly. I can't go out with ears like these.'

I looked at her ears, as instructed. The lobes were an angry red colour, tarnishing the appearance of an otherwise beautiful young Chinese woman. She was wearing gold earrings and they were encased in a horrid, yellow crust.

'I have come from Shanghai to study,' she told me with a strong accent. She spoke slowly and deliberately to ensure that I didn't miss a word or its meaning. 'My name is Ah Kum. I have been busy with my coursework during the week. I am sorry to trouble you late on a Tuesday evening.'

'Well, it's important that you've come to see me,' I answered, wondering what had happened to her ears and how best to treat them. 'As you see, we are packed out during the evening surgeries. Many patients can't make it during working hours, and this is the only time they can come.'

Ah Kum appeared to be a happy soul, despite her ear issues. She was very thin, although I suspected that this was just her natural oriental build; it didn't seem to be the painful thinness of an anorexic. She had a beauty about her, with gleaming black hair and an unmarked oval face with large, welcoming eyes. She must have been less than five feet tall in her flat sandals; Ah Kum was definitely one of my most petite patients.

'My name means as good as gold,' she chirped. 'Did you know that?'

I shook my head, probably with a puzzled look, and smiled. This student, in her late teens, still had a child-like quality about her and that innocence was reflected in those trusting, brown eyes. They opened wide, rarely blinking, as Ah Kum stood at my desk and then wriggled on to the chair opposite.

'You could be allergic to the metal in your earrings. It seems that the inflamed skin has become infected.'

'Oh, is that serious?' she asked, sounding worried for the first time.

'It would be best to remove your earrings,' I advised.

The Perils of Foreign Medicine

'I'm going to give you a prescription for an antibiotic cream to apply three times a day.'

Ah Kum was so elegant. All in one movement she removed and pocketed the earrings, accepted her written prescription, and tottered towards the door in a series of tiny steps.

'I suggest that you give the earrings a good clean – and any others you have worn recently. They are probably covered in germs from the infection.'

Ah Kum nodded, seemingly happy with my advice.

'It should clear up with the cream, but please come back if you have any more problems,' I said as she opened the door and closed it with a delicate click. That was that, I thought.

Well, that was that for a few days. Then the appointments diary on my computer showed that Ah Kum was due to make a reappearance on the following Thursday morning.

The day of the appointment came and I could see that Ah Kum was distressed. The earrings were still off but her lobes were inflamed and yellow; not a pretty sight. It seemed the antibiotic cream wasn't working – if anything, it was making matters worse and Ah Kum's face told me that she was having a miserable time trying to get her ears back to normal. There also appeared to be a white deposit on top of the yellow crust. I wasn't sure what that was – it could be the remains of the cream, which she insisted she was using. This hard-working, diligent and usually quite knowledgeable South London doctor was totally baffled.

I wondered if the bacteria were resistant to the antibiotic, so I took a swab to send to the lab. That would tell me which treatment I needed to use. I also told Ah Kum to stop using the cream and prescribed a different antibiotic to take orally instead.

'Be very careful,' I warned her. 'That pus is really infectious. Don't have contact with anyone until this is sorted out.'

Actually, the pus resembled impetigo, a highly contagious skin infection which causes sores and blisters. It's a common complaint and mainly affects children. It's caused by the staphylococcus aureus bacteria and spreads easily.

So, off she went, and I thought to myself – something really odd is going on here. In between appointments, I scanned my computer to check for similar cases. After a good trawl around medical sites, I was none the wiser about the white powder. But I had a suspicion that she would be back a few days later.

'Oh dear,' I gulped as a sad-looking Ah Kum walked over to my desk and sat in the patient's chair. 'We need to find out more about this.'

Her ears were much worse. They were dripping yellow pus and the teenager was wiping the mess away every five minutes to protect her clothes. I checked out the swab results from her previous visit. The cause of the infection was staph aureus, as I had suspected, and it was sensitive to the antibiotic, flucloxacillin, that I'd given her. The same applied to the antibiotic in the first cream. So both antibiotics should have worked and cleared up the infection without all this extra palaver.

Then I noticed there were more white deposits on her ears – and it didn't look like the cream I had previously prescribed.

'Have you been taking the antibiotics?' I asked gently. 'Or are you taking something else?'

'I have been taking the antibiotics,' Ah Kum said, firmly, without going into any more details.

I peered at her ears, close-up, to find out exactly what was going on. Those white deposits were really worrying me. I believed that she was hiding something. But why would she do that? What did she have to gain?

'You are going to have to tell me the truth,' I insisted. 'It looks like there is something else on your ears. What is it? If you tell me, we can solve your problems. Really, we can.'

Ah Kum began to cry, softly. 'I should have told you earlier. I am so sorry. I had an ear infection a few weeks ago and I used some special white powder. I brought it over from China – we believe in it and it is used for many ailments.'

'Do you have any with you?' I asked hopefully.

'Yes, here it is.'

Ah Kum pulled out a small food bag from her pocket,

giving me a glimpse of a white powdery substance, and then shoved it back inside her jacket as quickly as she could.

'Please do not take my powder,' Ah Kum begged. 'It is a traditional remedy from home. I must keep it with me at all times.'

I tried not to sound frustrated. 'Here is my advice: I have no idea what that white powder is but I suspect it contains steroids. They dampen down the immune system and that can make an infection worse. This appears to have happened in your case.'

'I need to keep using the special white powder. What is wrong with my special white powder?'

'Ah Kum, look at it this way. I am giving you anti-biotics which are tried and tested. They are safe, effective and ideal for fighting your type of infection. On the other hand, you have a special white power from an unknown source with unknown ingredients. Please use the antibiotics and steer clear of the white powder.'

My mini lecture worked. Ah Kum agreed to stop using the white powder. She fidgeted in her seat, continued to wipe her ears and then produced her jar of antibiotics. She had indeed been taking them as the jar was half full, but clearly she'd been applying the powder at the same time.

'I'd like to see you in a week's time.'

There were definite signs of improvement when I

next saw her and, finally, after about a month, her ears were virtually back to normal.

I was well aware that there was no way of knowing whether drugs bought from the Internet contained dubious ingredients. But this was the first time I had come across seemingly legitimate medicine, no doubt obtained from a legitimate source, which clearly contained substances that were potentially harmful.

It was not long before I was to have another misadventure with foreign medications.

'Doctor, I am feeling tired all the time. I don't seem to have any energy. I just want to go to sleep.'

She was a young lady from Thailand, probably in her mid-twenties. I guessed that she had married a Brit and moved to the UK to be with him. 'What's your name?' I began. 'I haven't seen you before – have you been in the UK long?'

'Kanya Ward-Jameson,' she answered in almost perfect English, proudly announcing the combination of her own name and that of her husband. 'We were married about two years ago. My husband Billy is a property developer with offices in the city. He is most concerned that I am tired all the time.'

'Your English is very good,' I observed. I thought to myself that it was going to make my life a lot easier. Trying to work out what was wrong with a patient who couldn't speak the same language as me was always a challenge.

'I prepared myself to come here by studying English at university and finding out about the British way of life. This is a great country. I wish I could enjoy it, though. I am just feeling so tired.'

'Are there any problems in your relationship?'

'I have no problems in my relationship,' she repeated matter-of-factly. 'My relationship is in very good condition.'

I probed further: 'Sleeping OK at night?'

'Sleeping OK,' again she repeated my words. 'But even if I have a good night's sleep, I am tired throughout the following day.'

'Do you have heavy periods?'

'No heavy periods.'

I was getting nowhere in record time. 'Are you a vegetarian?'

'Not vegetarian, and we have beef at least once a week. I thought you would ask about possible iron deficiency. I make Billy a dish called Thai massaman beef curry; I do not use any curry paste or powder. I put the beef in a curry pot along with the onion, bay leaves, potatoes, coriander, ginger and—'

'Sounds tasty,' I interrupted as she continued with the list of ingredients. 'But I can see that food has nothing to do with your tiredness.'

'Please, please, just give me some pills to make me feel better,' Kanya pleaded.

'We don't just hand out pills,' I answered firmly,

making sure that she understood my message. 'We need to find out first why you are feeling tired. Are you taking any medications?'

'No medications.'

'Do you have any other symptoms?'

'I just get a bit puffed, running for the bus. Apart from that I am OK.'

'You say that you sleep well enough. How much sleep do you get in a night?'

'Oh, I am always sleeping. It doesn't make any difference.'

I wondered if constant tiredness was the issue. 'Doctors sometimes abbreviate "tired all the time" – your problem – to TATT. The cause of TATT can be broken down into two main groups – physical and psychological,' I explained. 'The more information you give me, the better. I can rule out potential causes and seek out the reasons for your tiredness. And, more importantly, I can give you appropriate treatment.'

Our surgery is no stranger to cases of TATT and I could tell that Kanya was truly exhausted. On the physical side, lack of sleep is usually the main cause. This seems obvious, but many of my patients try to survive on six hours a night or less. For most people, that is simply not enough. An underactive thyroid – more common in women – can also be a cause of fatigue, and occasionally an overactive thyroid can have the same effect. Although an overactive thyroid makes people a bit hyperactive, it can also make them tired, particularly at the end of the day. Then there is lack of iron, which can lead to anaemia, which is another cause of severe tiredness. Just having low levels of iron in the blood can lead to fatigue – even if the haemoglobin level, the check for anaemia, is normal. This is more common in women who eat very little meat and do not make up for menstrual losses, especially those who have heavy periods. Type 2 diabetes is another culprit. This condition is more common in those who are overweight. In actual fact, tiredness may be the only symptom of their Type 2 diabetes. In older people, heart problems may be to blame and tiredness can also be a side effect of some drugs, such as anti-depressants, beta blockers (used to treat high blood pressure and heart disease) and some strong painkillers.

Often there are psychological, rather than physical, reasons behind the TATT symptoms. Depression, worry and anxiety drain the body. People who are in debt, or have job or relationship issues, can feel weary and, in turn, all that worry and stress leads to sleep problems.

Debt did not appear to be the root of Kanya's problems, though. As she sat in front of me, bleary eyed and yawning, I could tell that finances were not an issue – she wore blue designer jeans with a red top, all tightly fitting, and she wore an ornate wedding ring, as well as several other expensive rings and bracelets.

Kanya was plump but certainly not seriously over-weight. She was around five feet six inches tall – perhaps she had followed her homeland government's advice. A couple of days earlier, I'd read that boys and girls were being urged to drink a glass of cow's milk a day to increase height. Much of the milk sold in Thailand is the sweetened, condensed variety in cans. I haven't carried out any personal research, but the genuine article does contain calcium, vital for growing bones. I checked her pulse, and it was a little fast, at eighty-six beats a minute. That could have been caused by anxiety during her appointment. Blood pressure and pulse often rise when patients see their doctor.

The next step was to carry out blood tests to check her haemoglobin level for anaemia, although looking at her I thought this was probably not the problem. I also wrote out forms to check her iron level, sugar level and the levels of her thyroid hormones. The main hormone, thyroxine, is known as T4. A second hormone, triiodothyronine or T3, is usually present in smaller amounts. Both are produced by the thyroid gland in response to stimulation by the thyroid-stimulating hormone, or TSH.

Normally if the gland is overactive, T4 levels, and to a lesser extent T3 levels, go up and TSH levels go right down. The reverse happens with an underactive gland – the body produces more TSH to try to boost the thyroid gland into action.

The results came back a couple of days later. As expected, her haemoglobin level was normal, ruling out anaemia, and her iron and sugar levels were normal, too. But her thyroid results were confusing. Kanya's T4 level was normal, as was her TSH, but her T3 level was raised. This was bizarre; if the gland is overactive, then T4 levels should be raised as well and the TSH would be expected to go down.

I explained this dilemma to Kanya as best I could. 'Your results are a bit unusual.'

'It's not serious, is it doctor?'

I did my best to reassure her. 'No, it's nothing serious, but we need to repeat the tests, just to check the lab hasn't made a mistake.' I knew that occasional bizarre results are due to a problem with either the machines or the printer in the hospital laboratory.

But the results came through exactly the same as before. Not a lab error, then.

I phoned Kanya to explain that the next step was to arrange an ultrasound examination of her thyroid, to see if she had an abnormality in the gland which might account for the raised T3 level.

It was several weeks before she came back to me with the result, which had been given to her at the hospital.

'It says everything is normal,' she explained as she handed me the paper.

I read the report carefully and she was right. Her thyroid gland had a completely normal appearance on the scan, so why was that T3 level raised?

The Perils of Foreign Medicine

'I think we need you to see a thyroid specialist. They can do more tests and work out what's going on.'

'So, it is serious?'

Again I reassured her, as best I could, that her problem was unlikely to be anything nasty. I suspected she was worried she had cancer. If that had been the problem then her scan would have been abnormal.

I warned her that there was likely to be a two-month wait to see the specialist. I knew she would be worried during that time, but really there was nothing to justify asking her to be seen urgently. After all, her only symptom was tiredness.

I hadn't expected to see Kanya until after her hospital appointment, but the week before she was due to see the specialist, she came to see me with her husband.

Kanya looked tense and totally miserable. Her eyes were bloodshot and I wondered if she had had any sleep at all. Her husband, Billy, must have been in his late seventies. He wore a gold watch, gold bracelet, several gold rings and a slightly crumpled grey suit. The hair in his ears protruded, but I wasn't going to be the one to tell him.

'Hello, how are you? Are you any better?' I was hoping her mysterious tiredness had disappeared, although with her abnormal thyroid hormone results she would still need to see the specialist.

She didn't say anything. There was a short silence, broken by her husband. 'You need to tell the doctor about the pills you're taking,' urged Billy, talking to his wife. 'The doctor needs to know.'

This was new information to me. 'Pills? What are the pills for?'

Again, a silence.

'Tell her, Kanya. Remember that the doctor is here to help you.'

'Oh, they are nothing at all,' Kanya said defensively. 'I'm always trying to lose weight and the last time I was in Thailand I decided to try out some slimming pills.'

'I see,' I nodded, trying not to sound disapproving, but failing miserably.

Kanya was defiant. 'I went to a proper diet clinic in a proper hospital. The pills were prescribed by a reputable obesity expert.'

'Are you sure about this?' I asked both of them. 'There are many "backstreet" places and you just don't know what you are putting into your body.'

'There was nothing dodgy about the place,' Billy insisted. 'I went there myself to check it out. Everything seemed to be above board.'

I sensed that I was on the verge of a breakthrough, though. 'Please stop taking the pills, Kanya. I have no idea what they contain but it's possible that they are affecting the function of your thyroid gland. Stop them for a couple of weeks, then we'll repeat the tests, to see if anything has changed – and also we'll see if you feel less tired.'

The Perils of Foreign Medicine

Kanya's face screwed up, she glanced at Billy, and then she glanced at me. She stroked her chin and peered out of the window. She coughed politely and she stared at Billy once more. 'OK,' she agreed. 'But if it is nothing to do with the pills, may I start taking them once more?'

'You say they were prescribed by a proper doctor from a hospital, but we don't recommend pills for weight loss here. Not only that, I don't know exactly where they came from, what is in them or the effect they are having on your body. I'm a great believer that exercise and a proper balanced diet are the best way to lose weight. Would you mind bringing the pills in? I'd like to have them checked out.'

'OK, doctor, but please don't throw them away. This problem may have nothing to do with the pills. After all, they were prescribed by a doctor . . .'

I thought it best to delay her hospital appointment in the meantime. I suspected that I had found the cause of the problem and there was no point wasting NHS money on expert medical time and tests that weren't necessary.

Three weeks later, Kanya was back in the surgery. She looked a lot healthier and, when I checked, her pulse rate was back to a more normal seventy beats a minute.

'We need to do another blood test,' I explained, 'to see what's happened to your thyroid levels.'

'I have to say that I'm feeling a lot better,' Kanya smiled. 'Now I'm less tired, I've been doing lots of walking and keeping up a healthy diet. I was dreading stopping taking the pills – I thought I would gain weight. But, actually, if anything, my waist is smaller now that I've stopped them. By the way, here they are.'

I opened the brown jar, failed to understand the strange writing on the label, and emptied some of the contents on to the palm of my hand. They were small, brown, round pills. They appeared to promise health benefits and obviously delivered none at all.

The blood tests confirmed that her thyroid hormone levels were back to normal. In theory, higher T3 levels should have made Kanya feel more active, but in her case the opposite was true.

'I can see that the pills haven't helped me to lose weight at all,' she told me, looking happy at last. 'I just kept taking them because I had such faith in the Thai doctor. I can see that they just messed up the balance of my system.'

Kanya breezed off into the early evening hubbub and there was a gentle knock at my door, which suggested that Dr Naz was popping in for more discussions about our cases.

'What are they?' she asked as she saw the pills on my desk.

'Diet pills, apparently. Powder last time, pills this time – both seemingly prescribed by doctors. Not in this country, mind you. It is pretty shocking.'

I tried to get the little brown horrors analysed at the

local toxicology lab, but the service isn't available on the NHS. They are still sitting in my desk drawer. I'm sure they contain T3 and goodness knows what else. One day, I will find out exactly what they are.

CHAPTER FOUR

THREE WOMEN
AND A BABY

I have always maintained that I should have been a detective instead of a doctor. I spend much of my time gathering evidence, putting cases together and finding out who or what is responsible. There are always victims, too, and so a detective role would suit me down to the ground.

I made the suggestion to Fiona, our experienced and thorough practice nurse who has solved a few tricky cases herself. 'I'm in the wrong job, Fiona.'

She turned round and screwed up her face. 'No you're not!' She laughed out loud as she organised the family-planning leaflets in the waiting room. 'I think your work as a doctor suits you perfectly.'

'No, I should definitely have been a detective – you

have to be a bit like Sherlock Holmes to be a doctor,' I smiled. 'Perhaps there should be a role of doctor/detective?'

'Rosemary, you are talking nonsense,' Fiona yawned, tossing back her fiery red hair. 'Here I am, getting through the day after having both kids up coughing all night, and you're giving me a load of nonsense. Bah!'

'All right, then – what about the tragic case of Josh and his breathing difficulties? You pieced together the clues to find out what had gone wrong with his tablets and inhalers. Do you remember?'

'Yes, and you solved the case of that Roger bloke who was malingering,' Fiona agreed, coming round to my way of thinking. 'There was nothing wrong with him, in the end, and he really went after you when you discovered his ruse!'

'There you are,' I nodded. 'We solve mysteries all the time around here. Remember how you worked on all those MMR cases, trying to find out why numbers had dropped off,' I continued while the going was good. 'We also solved the case of the woman in her eighties who was still sexually active and spreading diseases here, there and everywhere. Wasn't she called Jean? I'm sure she was called Jean.'

'I can see that you have a point,' Fiona conceded. She gave me a thumbs up, picked up a load of necessities, and breezed off through reception into her treatment room for a series of children's injections. She had her hands full, in more ways than one, with follow-up checks on patients with diabetes and asthma.

I watched her close the door and knew that she would be greeting the people inside with enthusiasm and professionalism.

I settled down back in my office. A teenager – eighteen years old, to be exact – sat opposite my desk, chewing gum and scratching away at a spot on her neck. She was wearing skin-tight jeans tucked into ankle boots and a loose top. Her long, blonde hair didn't appear to be real; well, I suppose some of it must have been but I could see that there were extensions in a few places. She hadn't come for advice on her hair, though, and, as I prepared to take a few notes, Cheryl tugged at her blonde mane and explained her dilemma.

'I've missed my period,' she explained. 'It's been two weeks now. My friend says something must be wrong with my hormones.'

I handed over the box of tissues that always sits on my desk and looked at her sympathetically. 'Any chance you could be pregnant?' She seemed to have missed the most obvious cause of a late period.

'Don't think so – that's why it must be my hormones.'

'Which contraception have you been using?' I assumed that she was sexually active – it would be unusual to find an eighteen-year-old virgin in South London.

'We tried condoms, but he didn't like using them and he took them off halfway through. He said it was like sucking a sweet with the wrapper on.'

'So no protection, then,' I sighed, hearing an all-too-familiar tale. 'Have you never missed periods before?'

Cheryl wiped away her tears and collected her thoughts. 'I've probably been a day or two late, but never two weeks. I'm sure I'm not pregnant, though, so what other reason could there be?'

'Well, many medical conditions can lead to missed periods,' I answered carefully. 'I've come across reasons such as stress, a change in your weight and, yes, a hormone imbalance. But, from what you have told me, I think we need to start by doing a pregnancy test. I need a specimen of urine.'

'Do I need to do that first thing in the morning? Shall I wait until then?'

'No, there's no need to use an early morning sample. Could you do one now?'

I sent Cheryl off to the loo and told her to hand the specimen in to reception. I buzzed through to Fiona in the treatment room.

'Any chance you could do a pregnancy test for me? I would do it myself, only a couple of urgent extra patients have been added to my list and I could see them while I'm waiting for the result.'

As always, Fiona was obliging. 'Sure, Rosemary, no problem; though I might not be able to do it straight away. I've quite a queue of patients myself. I'll do it as quickly as I can.'

She buzzed back about fifteen minutes later. 'Rosemary, that pregnancy test for Cheryl – it's positive. No doubt about it.'

I called Cheryl back into my room.

She looked anxious, so I told her straight away. 'You are pregnant.'

'Really?'

'Yes, the tests we do here are pretty accurate. We can do another one on another sample if you like, but Fiona, the practice nurse, said there was no doubt about the result.'

'How far gone am I?'

'You said the first day of the last period was about six weeks ago? You'll actually have ovulated and conceived about fourteen days after that, but we always date pregnancies from the first day of the last period and expect it to last about forty weeks from then. So now you're about six weeks.'

Cheryl actually seemed relieved that she was pregnant and not suffering from a medical condition. 'At least I know now. I have a regular boyfriend and I am sure he'll be really pleased. He mentioned settling down the other day.'

'Oh?' I replied, surprised, as this would be fairly unusual in South London. I hoped that it was indeed the case.

'Yes. He's even bought me a ring. I'm not sure if it's a proper engagement ring, as he hasn't exactly proposed, but that doesn't matter. I know I only have a supermarket job, but we'll manage somehow. If we've got a baby we'll be able to get a council flat.'

Cheryl was wearing a gaudy ring on her middle finger. I wasn't sure whether now was the time to tell her that the lack of council housing meant a long waiting list for flats, and most new teenage mums still lived at home with their parents or in a room in a special hostel. That could come a bit later. I gave her some leaflets about looking after herself in pregnancy, a prescription for folic acid and vitamin D – both recommended in pregnancy – and referred her to the special antenatal clinic for teenagers. Cheryl left the consulting room – happy, it appeared, to tell her 'fiancé'.

The next day Mandy appeared in the surgery. She lived with her mother in a small block on the same council estate as Cheryl, close to the surgery. Around the same age as Cheryl, she wore similar denims, only this time with designer holes and rips.

'How can I help you?' I started.

'I'm pregnant,' she said straight away, nervously stroking her shoulder-length, brown hair. 'My period is about two weeks late. I've done a couple of pregnancy tests at home and they were both positive. I never imagined that I would get pregnant. I recently became engaged and my head is all over the place.'

'Were you using any contraception?' Pretty stupid question, I thought to myself. But I was prepared to give her the benefit of the doubt – it was possible she'd just accidentally missed a couple of pills, or a condom had burst.

'We were being careful.'

'What does that mean?'

'Well, he withdrew, you know . . .'

Oh dear. Despite everyone's best efforts, especially teachers in schools, local sex education had clearly failed again. Mandy had learned the hard way that the withdrawal method, with the man withdrawing from the vagina before orgasm, is a hopeless way of avoiding an unwanted pregnancy.

Although Mandy dressed like Cheryl, she was a totally different character. She showed no emotion, gave the briefest of answers and proved difficult to talk to. I established that she was studying hairdressing at the local college. I realised that a baby would delay her career and I knew plenty of young women who had dropped out of college altogether when they started a family.

'What do you want to do? Have you thought about having a termination?' It is often difficult to tell what women want to do about an unplanned pregnancy; it is important to broach the subject tactfully.

'Oh no. I'm sure my partner will stand by me. I hate the thought of having a termination. We'll manage somehow.'

'OK. I'll refer you to the antenatal clinic.'

'Why? Don't you look after me here?'

Doctor's Notes

I explained the system to her. 'There's a special team of midwives and other health care professionals at the hospital, and they look after teenage mothers-to-be. You'll have appointments with one of them, and also see an obstetrician – that's a doctor who specialises in pregnancy and birth. You'll also be offered antenatal classes, breastfeeding classes, and a whole lot more, especially as you are so young. They'll give you a lot of support at a difficult time.'

'Oh OK, that's all fine,' Mandy replied.

I wondered if she really had any idea at all about what life would be like with a baby. But it would have been unprofessional to try to persuade her to have a termination. And, unlike so many teenagers, she actually had a regular partner.

A few days later, a third pregnant teenager made an appointment at the surgery. As usual, Lizzy the receptionist had pointed all the young ladies in my direction, as I'm the doctor with a special interest in women's health.

Sitting in the chair this time was Chloe, aged seventeen, with a can of cola and a bag of crisps, a bag of shopping and a bunch of bananas, all threatening to fall on the floor. She clearly had either ignored or more likely not even seen the notice on the door about no food and drink in the surgery. Chloe, at nearly six feet, was a thin, willowy figure with short, close-cropped black hair.

'What can I do for you?' I asked, as the bananas lost

the battle for space on her lap and landed at the base of the chair.

'Sorry, I'm all over the place today,' she apologised, bending down to pick them up. 'I'm pregnant. Well, I think I am. My period is a couple of weeks late. My friend gave me a pregnancy test and it came out positive, I think.'

'Shall I do a test to be sure?'

'Oh yes, please.'

This time, rather than bothering Fiona again, I did the test myself, after Chloe had visited the loo to produce a urine sample. I explained to Chloe that if one pink band appeared on the testing strip, it was negative; two bands meant the test was positive.

We both watched as two pink lines appeared.

Her face fell. 'I'm unemployed and didn't really want this.'

Chloe did look 'all over the place'. She was confused, irritated, moody and happy all within a few minutes.

'Do you think you might want a termination? There's no need to decide anything in a hurry, but if you want to consider it I can give you some information.'

'I'll have to ask my boyfriend. I just don't know.'

She told me that her boyfriend had proposed to her, they hadn't used contraception and I could see that she lived close to Cheryl and Mandy. Although we often had pregnancies on the estate it was unusual to have three women, all around the same age, conceiving within a few weeks of each other. It was even more unusual for all the women to have a steady partner who had proposed and seemed keen on settling down. I was more used to women being abandoned by their boyfriends and having babies on their own.

Chloe came back to see me a couple of days later. 'I've thought about it and talked to my boyfriend. We'd like to go ahead and have the baby.'

I referred Chloe to the antenatal clinic and, once she was gone, I have to admit I sat at my desk for a few moments with my head in my hands. What was going on here? Why the sudden surge in teenage girls on the local estate abandoning contraception and presenting their fiancés with babies?

I tried as hard as I could to be open-minded but why couldn't these youngsters wait a bit and get their careers underway, with some money in the bank, before having a family? And, even more mysteriously, who were the young men who appeared so keen to get married? Surely they didn't all believe it was the quick way to escape from home and live in a council flat of their own?

All went quiet for several weeks, with not a peep from the pregnant trio. I knew that they would soon be under the caring wing of the local specialist 'teenage pregnancy' team of midwives. I was able to cope with patient after patient, fulfil my obligations to BBC Breakfast and the *Daily Express*, and still have time to look after my family.

Three Women and a Baby

The Rosendale detective agency was taking a short break from investigations.

One blustery South London Wednesday morning, I spotted pregnant teenager Cheryl on my list and assumed it would be a routine appointment. After all, this was her first baby and, sixteen weeks into her pregnancy, the chances were that she just needed some advice.

'I think I've got thrush,' were Cheryl's first words as soon as she sat down. 'In fact, I know that I have thrush. It can't be anything else.'

I told her that I wasn't too concerned. 'Thrush, which is caused by a yeast infection, is very common in pregnancy, because of high oestrogen levels. Are you itchy and sore, with a creamy discharge? Those are the classic symptoms.'

Cheryl just sat and looked at me, then admitted that didn't match up. 'I'm not really itchy or sore. I've just got a discharge. I assumed it was to do with the pregnancy but it's got a bit of a smell, so I thought I'd better come to see you.'

I needed to examine her, so asked her to get up on the couch. I discovered a greyish green discharge and an inflamed cervix. It didn't look like thrush at all. I took swabs to get an accurate diagnosis and wondered if she had chlamydia, which is quite common, especially in young people. If left untreated, chlamydia can spread to the womb and cause pelvic inflammatory disease, or PID. That condition causes infertility, miscarriage or ectopic pregnancy. An ectopic pregnancy results when a fertilised egg implants itself away from the womb – often in the fallopian tubes. In 2010, more than 186,000 people tested positive for the infection in England. Most were under the age of twenty-four.

Cheryl left after the examination and I told her that I would be in touch as soon as possible, but I urged her not to worry too much.

The following day Lizzy buzzed through from reception. 'It's a doctor from the microbiology lab at the hospital. He wants to speak to you personally. Says it's quite urgent.'

That meant an unusual or serious infection had been picked on one of the specimens I'd sent to the lab.

It was Cheryl's result. She didn't have chlamydia. She had gonorrhoea, or GC for short. Gonorrhoea infection is everywhere in South London and, with that in mind, I wasn't too surprised, even though it wasn't the result I had been expecting. I didn't relish the prospect of telling my patient. It wasn't something I could do over the phone so I asked Lizzy to get Cheryl into the surgery that afternoon.

It wasn't easy breaking the news to her. I had no idea at that stage where the infection had come from. It was possible she'd had it for ages as, like chlamydia, GC can hang around for months without causing any problems for the unfortunate carrier. I also had no idea about her partner and whether she'd had more than one.

Three Women and a Baby

'How come I've got the clap then? I've only had sex with my boyfriend for the past eight months. I had other boyfriends before that, but I was sensible and had STI checks at the local hospital.'

'With gonorrhoea there are sometimes no symptoms in men – although it would be unusual for a man to have it for eight months without any symptoms at all.'

I prescribed a large dose of antibiotics, assuring Cheryl that the baby would not be harmed. I insisted that she must tell her boyfriend, though, and that he should go to a clinic for tests and treatment.

'If he doesn't go to a clinic, you will just be re-infected. You really must tell him – to protect both yourself and others – though I admit it might be difficult for you to be concerned about other women at the moment.'

Cheryl reappeared a week later for repeat swabs and the results came back confirming that she was clear.

'Did you tell your boyfriend?'

'I – I – didn't,' she stuttered. 'How do you know that my fiancé, Ricardo, was to blame for the infection? Remember, I slept with other people before him. I want to marry Ricardo. This would just rock the boat.'

'You slept with the other men eight months ago. I agree it is possible you were carrying the infection silently all that time but, even if you are to blame, Ricardo will almost certainly be infected as well now. So he needs testing and treatment, too,' I said firmly.

I didn't want to remind her she'd told me she'd had

regular STI checks in the past. If that was true, it was likely that the infection had indeed come from Ricardo.

Cheryl stared at me defiantly. I could see that she didn't want to cause any problems in her relationship. She didn't want Ricardo to think she had given him something nasty; she also seemed to be blocking out the possibility that he had infected her. She had no intention of forcing him into a position of talking about his other activities. After twenty years of working in South London, I knew that whatever I said was unlikely to make any difference. Cheryl was in total denial.

Ten days later, Lizzy buzzed through from reception. 'I have a pregnant patient here with no appointment. She says she needs to be seen, and she'd like it to be with you, as you've seen her before. Can I fit her in as an extra, or do you want her seen by the duty doctor?'

I scanned down my surgery list. For once I wasn't running too late and only had a couple of patients waiting. 'I'll see her, but warn her that she may have a bit of a wait as she's being fitted in as an extra – unless it seems urgent. She's not in labour, is she?' I had memories of a scene a few years previously when a woman walked into the surgery unannounced and ended up giving birth in my consulting room within an hour!

'No, she's not in pain. She can wait,' Lizzy reassured me.

'I've got a bit of a discharge,' Mandy muttered as she came in. 'I think it's thrush.'

Like Cheryl, she had no itching or soreness, just some discharge; it was time for another examination. Mandy had the same greyish discharge. Not another one, I thought. I took swabs and advised her that I'd be in touch as soon as I received the result.

The following day, the microbiologist rang again. It was GC once more.

As before, Lizzy arranged to fit Mandy into the surgery as quickly as possible and I told her the news, as gently as I could, about the gonorrhoea. Again, she had been with the father of the baby for a few months before getting pregnant but she also admitted to having sex with an ex-boyfriend recently, too.

'I shouldn't have, I know, but I was a bit drunk. It was after I became pregnant, so I do know that Ricardo is the father.'

I clearly needed to remind her about the dangers of alcohol in pregnancy, but this was not the best time for that. It seemed too much of a coincidence that I had two pregnant teenagers, both with GC, and both 'engaged' to a man named Ricardo. Could it be the same bloke, I asked myself? But, if so, what was he doing proposing to two women at the same time? I had a sense of foreboding that one, or both women, would get hurt in the not-too-distant future.

'You must tell Ricardo and your ex-boyfriend,' I insisted. 'These men could be infected and pass it on.'

'No way, doctor. I can't tell them what I've got. I'll

tell them I've got a bit of an infection, but surely you can just give me a large supply of pills and I'll pass some on to them. No one needs to know exactly what the pills are for. They'll just take them.'

'That's not how it works,' I explained, somehow managing to remain calm. 'You must tell all the men you have slept with recently that they need a check-up.' I wondered if there were more than two. 'They need to have a clean bill of health before having sex with you – or anyone else, for that matter.'

'Look, doctor, I'm only going to sleep with my boyfriend from now on,' Mandy growled. 'So give me that double dose of pills and I'll be off.'

I wasn't giving up. 'It's impossible to tell exactly where the infection has come from so proper contact tracing has to be done. Not only that, but I can't give you pills to give to someone else. Apart from anything else, they may be allergic to them.'

'I just want to protect my relationship with Ricardo.'

I did feel some sympathy for Mandy. She felt guilty, but this wasn't the first time – and I was sure it wouldn't be the last – that I would come across a patient with multiple recent sexual partners.

Eventually, Mandy jogged out of the surgery with her prescription and my advice 'to tell all' ringing in her ears.

A couple of days later, Chloe rang asking for an appointment. According to Doreen she'd asked to be seen quite urgently as she was complaining about being 'a bit sore down there'.

This time, it was my turn to think that thrush could be responsible, especially when she said she was a bit itchy as well. But when I examined her, instead of seeing the thick, white, curdy discharge typical of thrush, it was grey with a green tinge. Oh no, not again, I thought to myself. I knew as I sent off the samples that they would probably confirm GC yet again.

An odd case of gonorrhoea is nothing unusual but to have three in as many weeks at my surgery is out of the ordinary – most cases are diagnosed at the local genito-urinary clinic.

When Chloe returned to receive the news, I tried to uncover even more of her story.

'Ricardo is my only lover. I haven't had sex with anyone else at all. He was my first proper boyfriend and he wanted to marry me. He said he loved me.'

'I see,' was all I could say. I was gobsmacked. Ricardo again! It looked as though he was the local Romeo, having unprotected sex with several women and leading to unplanned pregnancies and unwanted infections. That wasn't so unusual in South London. But I couldn't really believe he planned to marry any of them.

Unlike the others, Chloe quickly realised what had been going on. 'He lied to me! He said I was his first lover and he would never have sex with anyone else. I won't marry that little shit . . . but what am I going to do about the baby? I don't have a job at the moment, so things aren't easy.'

I arranged urgent treatment for the infection, told her that she must tell Ricardo and addressed the developing baby crisis.

'You are around twelve weeks pregnant,' I worked out. 'That is still early enough to have a termination, but you should have a few days to think about it. Just to be sure.'

'I honestly don't need any time. My mind is already made up. I can never trust him again. I am still young and would like a termination, please. I want it as soon as possible.'

I referred Chloe for the termination, but advised her that it was also important to clear the infection up first. If not, she was at high risk of developing pelvic inflammatory disease after the termination.

'I sense you don't really want to talk to Ricardo, but you really ought to tell him to get checked out. From what you have said, he's infected you and could go on to infect others as well.'

I wondered silently just how many more women this Ricardo character had infected. How many more were pregnant? Had he proposed to any others?

'Oh, Ricardo will find out soon enough. He'll be lucky if my dad doesn't murder him!'

'So he lives locally, then, does he?' I was curious.

'Oh yes,' Chloe hissed. 'Ricardo lives in the next

block with his parents. They're Spanish and Ricardo is a chef in a Spanish restaurant up in town. He is always going on about making tapas. Don't think I want to hear any more about Spanish food for a long time.'

Shortly afterwards a tearful Cheryl reappeared in my surgery. 'I've found out where my disease came from. There's been a lot of gossip on the estate. I met Chloe in the newsagents and we compared notes. I didn't know her before all this. We've been conned. Seems Ricardo was going to "settle down" with not just her and me, but there was at least one other girl as well. He's been sleeping with loads of other women, too. There is no way that I can have his baby. I need out of all of this. I'm sixteen weeks pregnant – is that too late for a termination?'

'Sixteen weeks is rather late for a termination, Cheryl,' I said. 'But in exceptional circumstances it is possible.'

Knowing the background, I thought her request was reasonable and I referred her to the termination service, knowing that they would also provide her with counselling. I felt that she had made the right decision. The situation clearly was not right for her to bring a baby into the world, especially with such a dubious character for a father.

That left Mandy still pregnant and determined to have Ricardo's baby. She returned to tell me her plan of action. 'I've found out everything,' she cried in my surgery. 'Word spread about what was happening but I could never agree to a termination. I just can't do it – I think I've felt the baby move. I'm clear of the infection and I just need to get on with my life with the baby when he or she arrives.'

A full eight months went past without any further incidents from this unhappy trio until a dreary, grey Monday morning. The rain hammered down as Doreen called through, 'I have a young mum on the line. Needs some advice. Could you talk to her?'

'OK, put her through,' I answered, taking a sip from the cup of lukewarm coffee on my desk.

'It's Mandy. My baby has a fever or at least he seems to have a high temperature. Also he is a bit sleepy and doesn't want his feeds. Could you come round?'

I could barely hear her for the rain pounding on the surgery roof.

'Anything over 37.5 degrees centigrade is a fever,' I told her. 'Could you bring him here? I can see him in about half an hour.'

'I would do, doctor, but I'm looking after my nephew as well as the baby. I don't quite know how I'm going to manage walking with the two of them in this weather. I can't afford a taxi.'

I wasn't planning any home visits that day but, as the estate wasn't far and I did have a car, I decided to go over at lunchtime. I advised her to give him some paracetamol in the meantime.

I knocked on the door of her flat and negotiated my

way past the clothes horses covered in baby clothes in the tiny hallway. Mandy was sitting on an old sofa in the lounge, cradling a sleeping baby.

I checked him over. His temperature was normal. 'He seems fine,' I observed.

'His temperature has settled with some paracetamol and he's just had a feed. I'm sorry to get you over. There was something else, though – I hope you don't mind, but could you come through here?'

Mandy led me into the bedroom where I was surprised to see Chloe and Cheryl sitting on either side of a double bed.

'Happy families,' Cheryl joked as I walked into the room. 'Word got around the estate and we heard about each other on the grapevine. Mandy did want you to check out the baby but we also wanted you to meet the man who is the cause of all of this and give him a hard time about sexual health.'

There was a sharp knock at the door.

'It's Ricardo,' Mandy explained, as she made the announcement. 'He always comes around about this time to see the baby. He doesn't know anyone else is here.'

Oh help, I thought: time for me to make a hasty exit. But it was too late.

As soon as he passed through the clothes horses, all hell broke loose. 'Cheater. Liar. You disgusting piece of filth.'

All the teenagers shouted at the same time and the stunned Spaniard stood open-mouthed as he surveyed the results of his romantic liaisons.

It was interesting to set eyes on the local lothario. I could see why the girls had fallen for him – he was tall, dark and, though I hated to admit it, quite handsome. He was also better dressed than a lot of the local young lads I'd seen around the estate. His jeans were not falling off to reveal his underwear and his jumper was clean. He did, however, reek of aftershave. He's handsome and he knows it, I thought to myself.

I realised I had been lured here under false pretences by three furious young women, but I could understand why. Ricardo's romantic arrangements were his own business but he was a walking health risk.

'What's going on here?' he looked at me accusingly. 'Who the hell are you? Did you set all this up?'

'No, Ricardo. I'm Dr Rosemary Leonard. I was asked to come and check on the baby.' He looked at me accusingly. 'However, now that I am here, I would also like to say that you must be more responsible about sexual health. These ladies have all had infections after sleeping with you. Please make an appointment at a genito-urinary clinic to get yourself checked out and make sure that you tell them about any sexual partners.' Silence. 'To your credit, I see that you are coming round regularly to check on your son, but you must agree that there has been a lot of confusion and heartache up until this point.'

Three Women and a Baby

'I see where you're coming from,' Ricardo mumbled sheepishly. 'Thank you for coming to see the baby. You are right about the sexual stuff, too. What I need to do is look after my son and make huge apologies to Mandy, Cheryl and Chloe.'

Ricardo began his attempts to explain everything. I felt that I had done my best for everyone in the flat. I walked away and left them to it.

Back at the surgery, Fiona was flitting between reception and her treatment room, coping with cuts and bruises. The recent downpour had brought with it a few stumbles and a confused pensioner who'd had a nasty slip asking for help.

'By the way, we haven't talked for a while about the case of the Casanova and the three pregnant women. Any update?'

'All investigations are complete. We have three victims and one culprit. We'll file it under "three women and a baby". Just call me Sherlock,' I laughed, as Fiona disappeared back into her treatment room to remove a young boy's stitches.

'Or Dr Leonard, I presume,' she answered as her door closed.

CHAPTER FIVE

METALWORK

As I drove into work one Monday morning, a paracetamol was beginning to have an effect on my slight headache. I hoped that the eight hours of surgery stretching ahead of me didn't bring anything too mind boggling. Just like anyone else, doctors have days when they feel a bit below par but, by the time I had filled up with petrol, listened to the Radio 4 news and parked, my headache had eased and I was able to focus on the day ahead. I greeted my colleagues and prepared to see a long list of patients, beginning with nineteen-year-old James.

'I don't need to ask what the problem is,' I told him, catching a glimpse of his swollen tongue. 'That looks like a real mess, James.'

'I know it is, doctor,' he tried to say but I could only just make out his words.

'Where did you have this done?' I gasped, surveying the damage inside the teenager's mouth. There was a stud through the end of his bright red tongue and I could see a bead of pus around the edges of the piercing hole.

'I had the piercing done a couple of weeks ago in the Far East,' James mumbled. 'I went out there during my gap year and fancied having it done just before coming home. Now I can hardly eat or drink and, as you can hear, I can barely talk.'

'I'm not the greatest fan of these piercings, James, and they are to blame for a lot of infections,' I pointed out. 'You can also suffer from chipped or broken teeth and even speech impediments. Was the equipment sterilised? What sort of place was it?'

James looked more than a little sheepish. 'It was some sort of backstreet parlour. I'd had a fair bit to drink and I can see now that it was a totally stupid thing to do. My mum has given me an absolute rocketing. She told me that I was too sensible for this, and that I'd let her down. She told me that she'd even heard of studs coming loose and being swallowed.'

I nodded in agreement, but didn't want to make him feel silly, which might put him off visiting the surgery in future. I also didn't tell James that bacteria under the tongue can spread like wildfire. Blood poisoning or toxic shock syndrome – fatal in some cases – poses a threat to anyone who takes these risks.

Metalwork

The only solution was to remove the offending stud, but this was a far from simple task because his tongue was so sore. Once I had finally managed to get the stud out, pus started to drip from James's mouth. I took a swab and, concerned about the piercing conditions in the Far East, prescribed high doses of two different sorts of antibiotics. I was trying to cover as many bases as possible to counteract a wide range of bacteria.

The results of the swab showed a mix of microorganisms but thankfully nothing too nasty. There are increasing reports of 'multi-resistant' bacteria emerging in the Far East; bugs that are resistant to all common antibiotics.

It took a full month for James' tongue to return to its normal size. When he returned for his final check-up, I gently tried to get home the 'keeping healthy' message once more. I was keen to find out if he planned any more fashion statements inside his mouth.

'Absolutely no way,' James said, without his previous mumblings. 'I've been reading a bit more about this. Did you know that dentists are worried about tongue studs?'

'Oh yes,' I replied. 'They can chip and damage your teeth. And, if the piercing isn't carried out cleanly and hygienically, people aren't just risking their oral health – their general health is at risk, too.'

James headed out of the surgery, on to his moped, and presumably off to college. After receiving my lecture, another teaching session was probably the last thing he wanted. And the last thing I wanted was another episode with metalwork – but that's what lay in store for me as the hours of daylight gradually disappeared and darkness enveloped us in mid-afternoon.

When Julia sat down in that heavily used patient's chair, it was soon clear it was yet another tongue-related problem. 'I can't talk properly,' the teenager grumbled out of the side of her mouth, giving a fair impression of a ventriloquist.

I peered inside her mouth. Julia had a metal device in the middle of her tongue. Pus was pouring out and the tongue itself was bright red and swollen. Through the pus, I could make out a bar made from cheap metal with balls on either end.

The advice for James was still fresh in my mind; I delivered the same facts to Julia, who appeared to take everything on board and looked quite miserable.

Julia didn't suit the ugly object in her mouth. She dressed like a normal sixteen-year-old and, rather surprisingly, hadn't had her ears pierced. The only other fashion accessories that I could see were tiny, sparkly studs stuck on to her brightly painted fingernails.

'Why did you have it done?' I asked. 'You don't seem to have any other piercings.'

'We were messing around in town and two of my mates had their tongues done. They dared me to do it, and here I am now with this horrible infection. They haven't had any problems, though.'

'They were fortunate,' I pointed out. 'I would guess

that the procedures – if you can call them that – were carried out under unsterile conditions. What sort of place was it?'

'We went to a jewellers a few weeks ago,' Julia explained. 'The person who did it was a young girl, to be fair. She clamped my tongue with some sort of forceps and put a needle through. I was hoping that my tongue would get better, but it's a lot worse now.'

'It's best if you let me know the name of the place,' I advised. 'It doesn't sound like the most professional operation. I think I should let the health and safety people know about it.' I had a closer look at her tongue. 'I'm going to try to remove that bar. The thing has to come out.'

Julia noticed my sterile gloves and I imagined that her previous experience hadn't been carried out in this carefully controlled environment.

'This is very different from the piercing place,' she muttered as I took a break to weigh up the situation. 'Oh, what a fool I am. I read that a lot of singers have these and even Zara Phillips had a tongue stud. I thought everything would be straightforward.'

'Well, we learn something new every day,' I answered, carefully poking around inside her mouth. 'I suspect those people didn't go to a Saturday temp at a backstreet jewellery shop.'

I tried hard to unscrew the two balls at either end of the flimsy-looking bar and both were reluctant to come off; I was amazed at the low build quality – they had rough edges. Even if the bar hadn't caused an infection, it would have made her mouth sore.

Then, success! Well, almost. I made some progress with the balls – off they came – but the job wasn't quite over. I wanted to remove the bar, gently and carefully, causing no more damage to Julia's mouth.

I had a rummage around in the store cupboard and found a pair of pliers. I knew that the piercing hole had started to close up. Slowly and deliberately, I grabbed hold of the end of the bar and eased it out. What a relief for all concerned.

'You're not out of the woods yet,' I warned Julia. 'That's quite an infection. I'm going to give you a course of antibiotics and you must take them as instructed.'

'OK,' Julia answered, still talking with a degree of difficulty. She managed a partial smile, obviously happy that the obstruction in her mouth had been removed.

'Come back in a week's time and we'll see what's going on.'

It took two weeks for Julia's tongue to return to its normal size. Even then, lemons and salt caused irritations and so she simply avoided them.

Two months after my impromptu piercing removal, Julia appeared for an appointment to ensure that her mouth had healed properly.

'The antibiotics have worked a treat,' Julia smiled, looking relaxed and relieved. 'I'm getting my ears done at a decent place but I'm going to leave the tongue alone. Is there anything I should look out for when I have my ears pierced?'

'Well, as it happens, large numbers of earrings are made from nickel, which is found in stainless steel and can cause an allergic reaction in the skin. At least once a month I see a pair of earlobes that are red and sore. The only solution is to take the earrings out and replace them with silver or, better still, gold; those two precious metals are far less likely to cause a reaction. So, check out the hygiene levels of the place when you get them done and the metal in the studs you choose.'

I had a close look inside her mouth. I could see some minor scar tissue around the initial wound, but nothing really to worry about. It's a normal part of the body's healing process.

Julia had a terrific sense of humour. 'Thanks for everything, doctor. I never really liked lemons anyway. They always left a sour taste in my mouth – even more so now!'

I joined in the banter. 'Well, I won't rub any more salt into the wound. Please come back if you have any more problems.'

Winter was beginning to embrace South London in its icy clutch and, as I drove into the surgery one morning, I spotted what could only be described as an 'alternative' vehicle parked nearby. It was an old VW camper van, circa 1973 or so, with a definite lean to one side and a fresh-looking lumpy red paint job. I could see a previous yellow coat shining through a collection of rusty dents.

I'm used to seeing a wide range of cars around the surgery area, varying from small-engined older models, driven by the numerous student patients, to sleek business cars. There are usually plenty of people carriers, too, used for ferrying kids to the local schools. But this was definitely something a bit out of the norm.

I parked beside this seventies throwback, wondering where it had come from and who would feel safe in the elderly machine. I deliberately walked past the lurching lump of scrap metal and checked it over. I was astonished to see that it was taxed for six months, which presumably meant that an MOT had been passed fairly recently. In the driver's seat I could see a hunched figure over the steering wheel. I checked my watch and saw eight o'clock clicking into place as Dr David's old green Jaguar drove into its usual spot, the tones of the *Today* programme on Radio 4 straining through the open window. Another look at the VW revealed the face of a young woman with multi-coloured hair. I braced myself for another full, varied and possibly bizarre day in my South London surgery.

With the doors about to open, the surgery was already starting to buzz. Fiona prepared her treatment room while Doreen and Lizzy tidied around their telephones. Naz had enjoyed a girls' night out, with all the trimmings, and the details were now being relayed to the rest of the staff. Dr David's consulting room was closed, as he avoided early morning chat and gossip when he arrived. He preferred to bury his head in his morning newspaper and post.

'Have you seen that rusting hulk of metal outside?' I asked Lizzy. 'Let's hope the patient inside is in better condition. Is she coming my way?'

'You do have a nine o'clock appointment for a cervical screening test with a new patient,' Lizzy confirmed. 'She's called Jenny. She called up a few days ago.'

I went up to my room and started up the computer. I checked there were no urgent letters or results that needed to be dealt with. At nine o'clock I called Jenny in, my first patient. The door swung open to reveal an extraordinary sight. I could see rings, more rings, shiny lumps of metal and a mass of tattoos. This chubby shape was encased in denim and even more metal attachments. She emerged from the waiting room with a wide, yellow grin.

'Hi, I'm Jen. It's short for Jenny. Ain't had a smear test before. Ain't got a clue about it, but all my friends say I need to get one done.'

I established that she was twenty-seven and had enjoyed sex with numerous different partners. I wondered what she used for contraception. 'Are you on the pill?'

'I took the pill a few years ago, but I kept forgetting, so I gave up on it.'

That was an all-too-familiar tale. 'Have you thought about an implant? It's put in your arm and lasts for three years. It provides excellent contraception, with no pills to remember.'

'I suppose I should,' she admitted. 'Some of the blokes wore condoms, but not all of them.'

When I started out as a GP, the mention of blokes, in the plural, would have had me raising an eyebrow. But not any more. It seemed that, for a lot of young people in South London, having sex was little different from kissing. I'd long since given up despairing about sex education and morals; it was just my job to try to stop them coming to any harm from their sexual activities.

From what Jen said, she was lucky not to have accidently become pregnant. I clearly needed to give her more advice about sexual health and contraception, but first I wanted to get her smear done. The more partners a woman has, the greater the risk of catching Human Papilloma Virus, or HPV, the virus responsible for cervical cancer.

As I chatted to Jen, I took in her appearance. Trying not to stare, I managed a sideways peek at her hair. There were blonde, pink and blue spikes everywhere. I'm sure there were hairy spikes on top of the hairy spikes. And then there was the metalwork: three rings in one eyebrow, four in the other, as well as a spike; a stud on one side of her nose; and a collection of different rings and studs in each ear. An impressive collection of silver-coloured bangles jangled on each wrist.

I realised it was, indeed, Jenny who had been behind the wheel of the ancient rusting hulk in the car park. 'Was that you I saw outside in a camper van?'

'Yeah, that was me, far too early for my appointment,' Jen confirmed. 'Ain't she a beauty? She was made in 1972 and has covered 500,000 miles – only a few by me. I just trawl round the festivals in her. We've been to the Isle of Wight, T in the Park, Glastonbury and all the others. Festivals are cool. I've seen Mumford and Sons, Kasabian, the Killers, the Foo Fighters and Deftones recently. Have you seen Rat Attack?'

Thanks to my sons, I was familiar with some of the names she mentioned and their music. But I had to admit that I hadn't actually been to see a group live in years. I suddenly felt rather old.

Jen fiddled with her spikes, folded her arms, and waited for instructions.

'Could you go behind those curtains and undress for me, from the waist down? Then get yourself up on the couch. Don't worry, the procedure won't hurt and I'll explain everything I'm going to do.'

Jen's examination is now called a cervical screening test but is often referred to as a smear test because of how it used to be carried out. The cells were removed from the cervix with a small wooden spatula, and not a brush as happens nowadays. In days gone by, the cells were smeared from the spatula on to a glass slide to be analysed. Today, the head of the brush on which the cells have been collected is placed in a small pot of preservative liquid. The brush can also be rinsed directly into the liquid as an alternative. The sample is sent to a laboratory where it's treated to remove any other material which may have been picked up, such as mucus or blood. The sample is then examined under a microscope to see whether there are any abnormal cells.

In all my years of practice I had never seen anything even remotely like Jen's metal collection. I should have guessed from her facial adornment that her body was unlikely to be a metal-free zone. Her tummy button had two rings, which wasn't so unusual. But it was when I asked her to remove her knickers that I had difficulty not registering surprise. As she opened her legs, I could see that a metallurgist would have had a field day.

Everything was pierced, and there were jingly jangly bits everywhere. I could see studs of all shapes and sizes, plus an extraordinary array of shiny objects. Her clitoral hood had been peppered with piercings. It was like a scrapyard down there, and was not a pleasant sight. I wondered about all the men she had mentioned; I would have thought that even a rampant male might think twice about making inroads in that delicate area. I longed to ask her why she'd had it all done, but didn't want to appear judgemental, or for her answer to make me feel even more ancient and out of date.

'What are you looking for?' Jen asked as I poked around. 'Do I have the Big C or something? My friends tell me that a smear test will check for all that.'

I needed to put her mind at rest. 'A smear test is a way of finding abnormal cells in the cervix – that's the entrance to the womb from the vagina.'

'Abnormal? I don't like the sound of that.'

'It's not a test for cancer,' I reassured her. 'Cervical screening checks the health of cells in the cervix and whether you are likely to develop cancer in the future. If so, they can be treated – so it's a way of preventing cervical cancer. But the vast majority of tests produce normal results.'

I wasn't keen on providing statistics during such a sensitive moment but I knew that one in twenty women showed abnormal changes in the cells of the cervix.

'Cosmic,' Jen said, nodding as I went to work with a clunk; this metallic maiden's accessories made a doctor's list of tasks more than a little difficult.

'Cosmic?' I spluttered as I assessed the problems confronting me. 'I haven't heard that word for a while . . .' Oh dear, I thought. Now I'm completely out of date with street talk. I really am ancient.

'Yeah, it's from the *Only Horses* programme. They're repeating all the old ones and that Del Boy says it all the time.'

I decided not to correct her on the programme title, as I feared it would only lead to more explanations.

Jen was a chatterbox on an unprecedented scale, though, and she kept up the banter. 'For some reason Trigger calls Rodney "Dave". I've never understood that. Del Boy calls him Rodney, but Trigger always gets it wrong.'

'I'm sure that it's all part of the programme,' I suggested, keeping an eye on the wall clock. I didn't want to overrun, as I knew that Doreen was fitting in a hectic timetable for me.

I went to work with the speculum. This is a medical tool for examining 'hard to reach' places; the name is Latin for mirror. The device looks like a big duck's bill with a screw mechanism to keep it open. You squeeze the handles and the 'duck's bill' opens up. The cervix is revealed, very carefully, allowing the doctor to carry out the test. The ratchet ensures that it can be locked in an exact position to make the job as easy and comfortable as possible.

I used a stainless steel speculum, which probably felt quite at home surrounded by all that metal. Plastic speculums are sometimes used. In rare cases these can break, but they are designed to ensure that any failure happens outside the patient!

'What are you doing now?' Jen asked as I ventured into the metal jungle.

'I'm just getting everything in place so that I can use a thin plastic stick with a brush at the end to gather some cells. It is very gentle and scrapes cells from the surface of the cervix. Then they're sent off to be tested in the lab.'

As I went about my routine business, disaster struck. All seemed to be going well; the 'duck's bill' was inside her vagina and I felt confident of success. However, Jen moved slightly and one of her metal rings became caught on the end of the ratchet screw. The device was stuck open, refusing to budge in any direction.

I tried and I tried, while trying not to make my efforts too obvious. I attempted a deft movement to the left with no success. I made a determined effort in the other direction – no success again. I wiggled and jiggled, ever so slightly, but the ring remained firmly in place, locked on to the ratchet of the speculum. Del Boy would have called me a plonker.

Jen could tell that a bit of metal on metal was going on and that it was far from ideal in her private area. 'Is everything OK? You seem to be doing an awful lot of fiddling.'

I decided honesty was the best policy. 'Rings and studs everywhere, and they're disagreeing with my equipment,' I said calmly, but I was feeling far from calm. 'I'm just sorting it out now.'

Well, I was trying to sort it out. I was sweating profusely and gently trying to ease the stuck speculum out of the embedded ring. I thought about fetching Fiona or Naz, who could have provided a much needed extra pair of hands. However, my own pride kept me at my post.

'Don't stress out,' Jen advised, realising that I was in a slight panic mode. 'What's the worst that can happen? It ain't gonna kill me.'

Well, that was true, I reassured myself. However, one wrong move and the ring could have torn through her labia. That was a far from ideal scenario and not one that I fancied having to explain or justify.

After a bit more gentle jiggling, the ratchet finally emerged from the ring of rings. I examined the damage – nothing apart from some slight bleeding. I sorted that out, fulfilled the rest of the requirements of the test and breathed an enormous sigh of relief.

'Is that it, then?' Jen asked eagerly as she clambered down from the couch. 'Are there any diseases down there? Do I have the Big C? Is anything abnormal?'

'You'll have the results in two or three weeks. Remember that this is just a test for abnormal cells. Most results show that everything is normal. You should get a letter in the post to your home and we'll also get a copy here.'

'I'm off travelling again soon, so could you call me if anything's wrong?'

We always chased up on abnormal results, anyway, so I reassured her that the surgery would be in touch if anything was amiss. I also gave her a handful of leaflets about contraception and asked her to make an appointment to come back to see me as soon as she could.

I wondered when Jen had last had a wash. She hadn't

come for advice on hygiene but I could tell she had a relaxed attitude to cleanliness, judging by her dirty fingernails. I imagined that she lived in her van a lot of the time, but it really was none of my business.

Despite the problems during Jen's test, I was pleased that she had come forward for screening. Women between twenty-five and forty-nine should be tested every three years; older women are invited to have tests every five years. I was also really grateful that she'd been so co-operative about my difficulties with her rings and the speculum.

Around three weeks later, Jen's envelope with the results arrived at the surgery. I really hoped that everything would be in order. As I prepared to open the envelope, I recalled the various possibilities: if your results are normal you don't need to do anything. Just wait until your next test is due. The results may come back as 'inadequate'. This means that the test couldn't be read properly. In these cases it is possible that too few cells were collected, or the sample was contaminated with blood or mucus. In older women the cells could be dry and inflamed due to lack of oestrogen. Then there is 'borderline'. This occurs when there are very slight abnormal changes in the cells, but they are still almost normal, and treatment may not be required. In this case you will return six months later for another test to find out exactly what is happening. With many patients, the follow-up result is back to normal.

Doctor's Notes

The one result I don't want to see, of course, is 'abnormal'. The changes in the cells could be mild, moderate or severe, depending on the degree of abnormality present. All three categories mean that pre-cancerous cells are present, but it does not mean that you have cancer, or that the Big C, as Jen put it, is heading your way. Mild changes need to be monitored and re-checked six months later as, like 'borderline', everything reverts to normal. But a second abnormal smear, or anything moderate or severe, needs more investigation. Left untreated, the cells could develop into cervical cancer.

If further investigation is needed, you will be referred to a special gynaecology clinic. This specialist will carry out an examination known as a colposcopy, using a microscope called a colposcope. This determines whether or not you need treatment to sort out the abnormality in the cells.

I read Jen's test results carefully. The letter said that Jen had severely abnormal cells. Without treatment she was at high risk of these developing into cervical cancer.

I decided to ring Jen straight away. I did not want her travelling around the country in her van and not receiving her result. 'Hello, it's Dr Leonard. I have your results here. Are you in London? Would you be able to pop in to see me?'

'What's wrong?' she asked. 'Is there a problem?'

'Well, there is some abnormality and so we need to have a chat.'

'Tell me now,' she insisted. 'Go on – spill the beans.'

'You need to have some more tests,' I explained. 'Please come in if you can.'

I checked my appointments diary and managed to fit her in that same afternoon. I probably go overboard sometimes with these cases and burn too much midnight oil, but that is how I operate. I like to know I've sorted someone out properly, even if it cuts into my personal time.

There was no wide grin when Jen appeared at the surgery this time. She looked worried and sat down without saying a word. She wanted to hear the exact details from me; I could hardly deny her that service.

'I need to refer you for colposcopy to find out the extent of the problem. The doctor will then take a biopsy to confirm the smear diagnosis. After that, you will be called back for a LLETZ procedure – this is where heat is used to destroy the abnormal cells.'

'I don't like the sound of that colposcopy thing,' she moaned. 'I bet it's painful.'

'Well, it isn't painful; although, being honest, it can be a bit uncomfortable. Try and relax as much as you can; that will help. On both of your visits you'll lie on a couch with your legs in stirrups. The cervix is painted with dilute acetic acid to highlight any abnormal areas. The colposcope magnifies the view of the cervix and surrounding area, so the doctor knows which cells to target.'

'OK. Better that than the Big C.'

As I wrote the referral, I couldn't help thinking about the doctor at the hospital. He or she would discover the array of metal objects during the examination. What would they make of it all, I wondered? Would they, like me, make a hash of the examination?

A couple of months later, Doreen poked her head around my door. 'The lady with the abnormal cells – the one with all those rings and studs – just called. Could you see her tomorrow?'

'Of course,' I said, knowing that I had a jam-packed day but, at the same time, keen to find out how Jen had got on.

'Here I am again,' she announced. 'I seem to be your resident patient.'

'How can I help?'

'I'm really sore down there,' Jen complained. 'They said I might get an infection of the cervix after that LLETZ treatment. Could you have a look?'

My heart sank. The last thing I wanted was another close-up view of the metal jungle. I braced myself, gritted my teeth and prepared for a repeat performance – hopefully with no entanglements this time.

I pointed towards the examination couch and Jen slipped in behind the curtain without a word. She was getting used to examinations in her intimate areas.

Metalwork

Off came the underwear and, surprise, surprise, there was no metal to be seen; there was not a single stud, ring or shiny accessory anywhere on her lower body. I also noticed an improvement in hygiene, which even extended to her now brightly painted nails.

'Things have changed a bit. You've removed the apparatus down here.'

'Yes, they all had to go,' Jen laughed. 'You got into a bit of a tangle last time. The hospital doctor got in an even bigger mess, trying to get that speculum thing in and out, if you know what I mean.'

'I know what you mean,' I nodded, grinning to myself. So it wasn't just me who was a bit incompetent when the genital area had extra adornment.

'Ain't fair on the doctor and also it was pretty sore for me. And when they started talking about heat treatment I got worried about the metal getting hot. So I had them removed. They were all gone by the time I went for that LLETZ treatment.'

I was so relieved. 'I see. I wondered whether the doctor had asked you to remove them. It certainly helps with this type of examination.'

In the metal-free environment, I was able to see everything very clearly. Although Jen's labia were enjoying a stud-free existence, they weren't back to anything like normal. The weight of the metal had stretched the skin, so her labia were much longer and much more uneven than usual. And it wasn't her cervix that had become infected – it was one of the piercing holes. Jen's left labia minora (the 'inside flap') was red and swollen. I was amazed that she was wearing tight denim 'jeggings' and suggested she would probably find tracksuit joggers more comfortable. 'A skirt,' I said, 'would be even better. You've got a slight infection here. It's best if nothing rubs against this area – it will just make it more sore. It should clear up without any problems, though. I'll prescribe antibiotics.'

So Jen waltzed off towards her elderly camper van, where twenty years of old oil was leaking all over the place and that was the last I saw of her. I doubt that her labia will ever shrink back to normal after all that stretching from the metal. Sooner or later I expect to see her back at the surgery asking for labiaplasty to reshape them. She won't get that on the NHS as it's a cosmetic procedure – and an expensive one at that – so she'll need to find a goldmine, rather than her scrapyard, to pay the bill!

As the day drew to a close, I toured reception and decided we needed more information about cervical screening to be displayed.

'Have we any more leaflets?' I asked Doreen and Lizzy as I filed the last of my paperwork. 'We've got a strong message to deliver. And I want to get it out there as soon as possible. We need a smear campaign to keep all our lady patients checked and healthy.'

Metalwork

As I tidied up, I also thought about Jen and her passion for music festivals. I had never listened to some of the bands she mentioned. I couldn't believe that things had changed so much over a few years. With the surgery door locked just after 6.30pm, I was able to test my colleagues' musical knowledge.

'David, do you know who Mumford and Sons are?'

'Sounds like a removal company. Are they over Bromley way?'

'Nil out of ten,' I marked Dr David on his knowledge. 'What about The Saturdays?'

'Do you mean the day of the week? No, Rosemary, I've not heard of them. But The Rolling Stones are still going, aren't they? And I'm a big fan of Shirley Bassey.'

'You are even worse than me! You are about fifty years behind the times!'

'Yes, you should keep up to date,' Lizzy and Doreen chipped in. 'It would help you to bond with your patients . . . Although, maybe not the elderly ones!'

A few weeks later, as Dr David's Jaguar eased its sleek lines into his favourite parking spot outside the surgery, I heard some extraordinary sounds coming out of his open windows. I walked over to his car and saw him tapping on the dashboard while a familiar tune blasted through his loudspeakers.

'That sounds like Petula Clark,' I told him. 'You *are* stuck in the sixties!'

'Wrong about the sixties,' he corrected me with a

smug grin. 'Yes, it is Petula Clark but she is singing "Downtown" with a modern outfit called The Saw Doctors. I've switched to Radio 2. Now I can enjoy my old tunes with a new twist. I also have that old Welsh wizard Tom Jones with The Stereophonics. And he's been singing with The Cardigans. See? I can have the best of both worlds.'

'Well, it is a start,' I conceded.

The beaming Dr David had really done his research after his ribbing. 'Did Max Bygraves ever do anything with those Stone Roses? I need to build up my stunning new music collection.'

'Subject closed,' I muttered and decided that all future discussions would be on a strictly medical basis.

'What about Abba . . . ?' Dr David's voice tailed off as I bolted into the surgery.

CHAPTER SIX

I DIDN'T WANT TO LOOK LIKE THAT!

'I just want to hide away,' Amina whispered softly, hiding her head in her hands. 'I can't even look you in the face, Dr Leonard. My confidence has gone and I have nothing to look forward to.'

I handed her the box of tissues that always live on my desk. 'What on earth has happened? How can I help you?'

Amina's face remained hidden behind her hands and tears appeared between her fingers. Amina had always taken pride in her appearance. She was in her mid-thirties with smooth, dark, glowing skin and an overall sophisticated look. Her gold earrings, bracelets and rings oozed quality. She was wearing a loose cashmere jumper, well-fitting, tapered, black trousers and plain, black court shoes. Everything appeared to be elegant, except for her demeanour.

Amina's straight, jet-black hair always gave the impression that it had been styled a few minutes ago. I remembered that, from our previous appointments, her family came originally from the Swahili coast in East Africa. She had no interest in religion, saw herself as English through and through, and held down an executive role with a well-known insurance company.

Amina was still holding back about her reason for coming to see me. 'Why are you so distressed?'

Amina answered, removing her hands from her face at last. 'I'm in a total mess.'

'In a mess?' That usually meant an emotional problem. 'What's happened? I think it would help both of us if you got whatever is bothering you off your chest.'

'That's my problem,' Amina whispered. 'That's my problem.'

'Your problem?' I asked, no doubt with a puzzled expression. 'I'm not with you.'

'You mentioned my chest, and you were just using a turn of phrase,' my anxious patient explained. She pulled herself together a bit and her tears dried up, leaving light traces down her cheeks. 'It was rather apt, though, because my chest is the problem.'

'Let's start at the beginning,' I said, slowly and deliberately. 'Let's get the whole story and we can decide on a way forward.'

I Didn't Want to Look Like That!

'It is a horrible story,' Amina grimaced. 'You won't want to hear it.'

'Yes I will, Amina,' I assured her. 'Whatever your problem is, I promise to do my best to help you. That's what I'm paid for. It's my job.'

'OK.' She took a deep breath. 'I had what they call breast augmentation at a private clinic in the West End. Breast implants. It's been a disaster from start to finish.'

'What happened?' I couldn't see the exact shape of her breasts through her sweater, but they certainly looked rather big and out of proportion to her otherwise small frame. I wondered if they had ended up larger than intended.

'My breasts are so sore. I can't wear a bra at all – it hurts too much.'

'I need to have a look.'

'But it's so embarrassing. They are such a mess.' Tears welled up in her eyes again.

'Don't worry about being embarrassed,' I reassured her. 'I'm sure whatever has happened I will have seen far worse.' I fervently hoped this was true.

As she prepared to remove her blouse, Amina told me that both her breasts were painful, uneven and lumpy after the operation. 'I rang the clinic, but they weren't interested. They said it was most likely just normal swelling from the operation, and that it would settle down in a few days. They just said if I was worried I could always go and see my GP. I waited a few days, hoping it

117

would get better, but it hasn't – it's got worse.' I was horrified to hear the details. 'It's nothing like the clinic led me to believe. They sent me home with a sheet of paper with instructions. No one actually came and talked to me about post-operative care or anything like that. After I paid the money, they seemed to lose interest.'

Amina slipped off the sweater, folded it and arranged the garment neatly beside the couch. She lay down and I could see immediately why she was so upset. Both breasts looked not only huge, but puffy and lumpy. Worse still, they weren't the same shape or size. The left one was higher than the right one. Not only that – the lower half of her right breast was red, sore and swollen. The cut underneath her breast, where the implant had been inserted, was badly infected.

It looked like a real botched job, but it wasn't going to help her, in her current state, to say so. Neither did I want to tell her that the skin looked so stretched around the implant that there was a high chance the wound would break down. I didn't like the look of it at all.

'It appears the incision – that's the cut where the implant was inserted – in your right breast has become infected,' I explained. 'You need some antibiotics, which I'll prescribe for you.'

'And will that help them when they're looking so odd? The left one feels lumpy and it looks higher than the right.'

I Didn't Want to Look Like That!

'Both the breasts are swollen and puffy. It looks as if you have reacted in some way to the implants. That, hopefully, will decrease over the next few weeks, and they will look different once this infection has settled, too. Give it some time.'

I tried to be reassuring, but I was dubious whether they would ever look symmetrical. It looked to me as if the implants had been put in different places.

'I wish I'd never had this stupid operation in the first place,' Amina admitted. 'Looking back I was a size ten with adequate breasts – 34B – for my shape and size. But my head was turned when I saw an advert in a magazine. It had impressive "before and after" pictures, and the woman's breasts were amazing. I wanted to look like that.'

I longed to ask Amina whether she thought it would make her more attractive to men, or whether it was done to please herself, but this did not seem the right time to delve into her motives. 'Do you still have the advert?'

'Yes, here it is,' Amina replied, producing a crumpled piece of paper from her handbag. 'Look, they have pictures of women with gorgeous breasts. I wanted to have a figure like that.'

I doubted whether many of this clinic's victims – and I reckon most of them were victims, rather than patients – enjoyed the glamorous 'post-op' look. I had come across other disastrous cases in the cosmetics industry and Amina was the perfect example of how procedures could backfire with horrendous results.

I opened up the crumpled advert and spread it on my desk. The 'before' picture showed a glum, slim woman – in her mid-twenties, I would say – with small breasts contained in a skimpy bra. Beside it, in the 'after' picture, the same lady was grinning from ear to ear, and her breasts seemed to be more than twice the size. I felt sure the photograph had been digitally altered to make it look more appealing. The 'after' picture certainly showed a large cleavage, if that was what a woman wanted. The advert described how different cup sizes could be obtained; it said that, for a limited period, a special deal was on offer.

'I fell for it hook, line and sinker,' Amina sighed. 'You must think that I am so gullible. I didn't even check out the clinic. Well, that's not entirely true. I read some reviews and they were all excellent. But I realise now I have no way of knowing if the reviews were genuine – they could have been planted by the company. I was so desperate to have larger breasts that I forked out thousands of pounds.'

'It might be best if I take some notes,' I suggested. 'What happened when you went to the clinic for the first time?'

'Well, they started with some sort of counselling from a young woman in a nurse's uniform. I think she was Eastern European. I have no problem with that at all. What I have a problem with is that, looking back, I reckon that she had no qualifications at all. I should have clicked at the beginning because, when I asked her questions, she had to look at her computer to know what to say. And, at one stage, she even disappeared and came back with the answers. I imagine that she was looking things up on the Internet, or asking someone else, and then coming back with the right information. What a con.'

'Who carried out the operation?' I asked, still making some notes.

'I'm not sure and that is one reason why I am so unhappy,' Amina complained. 'When I went in a few days later to have the operation I was seen by a young doctor. His English wasn't too good and so everything was rather vague. I had the general anaesthetic – I don't know who gave me that either, because I didn't meet the anaesthetist beforehand. You can see I have no idea who carried out the actual operation. It could have been the confused nurse person, for all I know.'

Amina's comment lightened the mood. The thought of the nurse, or secretary for that matter, manning the reception and then nipping into the operating theatre to carry out a bit of cosmetic surgery made me smile. The thought made Amina snigger, too, and I was delighted that she'd calmed down a little.

'It just shows you how amateur the clinic was. No one knew very much about anything and I was such a fool,' Amina reflected. 'I thought my breasts were small for a black woman. I saw those pictures of voluptuous models and I wanted to be like them. I read all the forums and the success rate was high. The only issue people recorded was something known as keloid scar tissue, which apparently occurs more often in people with darker skin.'

'Yes, that's right,' I said. 'It's a hard, smooth, pinkish growth at the exact point of the injury. You don't appear to have any of that, though.'

'I'm so sorry to have to come to you with this. It's all my own fault.' Tears started to well up again in Amina's eyes. 'I can't seem to think straight. I feel so stupid. And now I realise I don't even know what type of implants have been put in. I should have asked about that, and didn't . . .'

'Don't berate yourself,' I urged. 'You were drawn into this because of the advertising and I can see why. Hopefully the antibiotics will deal with the infection and, in a week, your breasts will look much better. Come back and see me then. Meanwhile, would you mind leaving this advert with me? I'd like to try to find out a bit more about this clinic.'

'Have you ever seen anything like this?' I asked Naz when she popped into my room to raid my supply of speculums. 'This "before and after" stuff, and the information about the operation is appalling.'

'Yes, it is appalling,' Naz agreed, rummaging around in the box to find the exact size of speculum she needed. 'I saw another advert similar to that in the back of a women's magazine the other day. It said that breast implants could be inserted during a lunch hour, under local anaesthetic, for £4,500.'

'What, like having your hair done? Just get your boobs enlarged instead of a blow dry? I've heard of people having facial fillers done in their lunch hour, but not a boob job.'

She nodded and tapped on my computer. Sure enough, the advert appeared, backing up everything Naz had said. I shook my head in disbelief, Naz made a speedy exit and I prepared for my next patient.

Just over a week later, Amina appeared at the surgery again in tears.

'It's worse,' she explained. 'The cut on my right breast has burst open, and now it's oozing.'

I eased her gently in the direction of the couch and prepared for the worst. I closed the curtain, while Amina slipped off her jumper. She had stuck a large piece of gauze over the bottom half of her right breast, but I could see it was already soaked with yellow, blood-stained fluid. As soon as I removed the gauze, I saw that the wound had indeed burst open.

'Will this ever heal? Will the implant fall out?' Amina asked me anxiously.

I surveyed the mess. The edges of the cut were being stretched by the large implant, and gaping at least an inch part. I thought it unlikely that it would heal without further surgery to pull the skin together. But that couldn't be done until the infection had been sorted out, or it would just break down again. Not only that, but the wound needed careful professional dressings to try to keep it as clean as possible. I explained this to Amina.

'Please just stay there a moment,' I told her. 'I'd like a chat with the practice nurse.'

Fortunately, Fiona had just finished applying dressings to an old lady who kept falling from her mobility scooter. The lady left the surgery with her leg neatly bandaged and I seized my opportunity.

'Fiona, do you have a moment? I have a patient called Amina who's had a disastrous breast operation. If you could possibly dress the wounds, I'll prescribe another course of antibiotics.'

'Yes, of course,' Fiona answered, clearing her desk and rearranging her room after a frantic morning. 'I'll be ready in about five minutes, if she'd like to come through then.'

I couldn't send Amina back into the waiting room with her breast dripping pus, so I chatted to her while we waited.

'I should have left my breasts the way they were,' she admitted. 'They were just on the small side. Now they are an unsightly mess and I will never be able to have a relationship again.'

'I thought you were in a relationship?'

'Well, I did have a boyfriend,' Amina said, tearfully. 'But we broke up about six months ago. I thought it might help me to find another man if I had bigger breasts.'

'Did you last boyfriend ever say anything about your body?' I gently probed. I would have found it easier to understand her decision to have surgery if he'd suggested that her breasts were too small.

'Not exactly, he just said he didn't think we were suited. I don't think he fancied me any more. But now I realise that it probably had nothing to do with my boobs . . .'

Amina made her way to the treatment room and emerged a few minutes later, professionally patched up with Fiona's dressings.

I caught up with Fiona at the end of surgery.

'I cleaned everything up and applied the dressings as well as I could,' she told me, 'but her operation has been an utter disaster. I would like to know who put those implants in. They should be struck off. Everything about the job looks amateur. I'm not convinced that the breast will heal, you know.'

I nodded in agreement.

'When she comes back for her next appointment,' Fiona continued, 'I'll check the dressings, so if you could give me a knock, please.'

Amina returned to the surgery after finishing the course of antibiotics and I wondered what lay in store for me in the examination room. Surely, I thought, the antibiotics would have worked this time. No such luck.

After Fiona had changed the dressings, I decided I had to lay it on the line for Amina. The truth couldn't be avoided any more. 'This wound isn't going to heal on its own. It's being stretched too much by the implant. And the skin is now so scarred, I don't think even a qualified surgeon will be able to make a good job of it. I think the implant in your right breast will have to come out.' Her face fell. 'It's the only way, I'm afraid. I can refer you on the NHS, but they won't be able to do it straight away – it doesn't count as an emergency.'

'That bloody clinic should help me out with this.' I was surprised at Amina's language. 'It's their fault that I'm in this mess. Maybe I should threaten to sue them.'

'If you could wait for the NHS, at least you can be sure you are in good hands . . .'

'I can't keep walking round with a hole in my breast like this. Surely they couldn't botch up taking the implant out?'

'Well, if you do go back to that clinic, please make sure that you know exactly who is going to be doing the operation this time, and what they plan to do. Please. And give me a call if you need any advice.'

The next day Doreen caught my attention as I walked through reception after a comfort break.

'I have a woman on the phone about her breast operation. It's the lady you saw the other day. She's rather anxious to speak to you.'

I Didn't Want to Look Like That!

'Put her through,' I said, entering my room and hoping for some good news.

'It's bad news, I'm afraid,' Amina muttered. 'They say that, despite all the complications, I will have to pay for a second operation.'

'What?' I blurted out into the receiver. 'I would have thought the clinic must take some responsibility for this? Did you threaten to sue them like you said?'

'Yes, but it didn't make any difference. It was that same women on the phone, the one who "counselled" me – ha ha – in the first place. She read out the small print on the agreement. When I signed for the original operation, I signed for a "cut-price" deal. The agreement covered just one operation. It excluded any complications, follow-up care or anything else.'

'They don't seem to care,' I concluded. 'I suppose they are within their rights, as you've signed the form. But you would think they would help out as it has gone so wrong.'

'I am amazed, too, but the woman insisted that I would have to pay.'

I stared at the advert in anger when the call was finished. I wrote out all the details for the local NHS breast clinic, thankful that I had recorded all of Amina's problems. It meant that I could provide them with chapter and verse. I just hoped they could help her out as soon as possible, but dealing with an implant 'gone wrong' was nowhere near as important as dealing with breast lumps that could be cancerous.

The NHS clinic saw Amina a couple of weeks later. They said that they could remove the implant from the infected right breast, but would not cover the cost of removing the implant from her left one. They said she would have to pay for that. It did seem unfair, but I could see their point. She didn't actually need the left one removed, especially as she might decide, eventually, to have another implant in the infected breast.

I felt that I had done everything possible to resolve the case. I wanted to give the private clinic a piece of my mind about the lack of follow-up care, and their general attitude, but kept my powder dry.

'Well, here I am and I am ready to go straight on the couch,' Amina said when she arrived to see me for a check-up after the second operation. 'I think I know the ropes by now.'

I studied the damage to her right breast. The result of the initial operation and then removal of the implant had left the breast puckered, misshapen and not attractive at all. And, of course, Amina had a totally lopsided appearance as her left breast was still huge because of its implant.

'You couldn't make this up,' my distressed patient mumbled. 'I don't know whether to have another implant on the right side, or have the left implant out and go back to square one. This has taken over my life. That clinic should be closed down.'

I Didn't Want to Look Like That!

'Certainly they should be controlled better,' I agreed. 'But don't go making any quick decisions about your breasts. Wait a few more months. You've been through so much that you may want a break from all this. Take as much time as you need to make a decision.'

After a week or two of thinking, Amina was back in the surgery with her mind made up. I braced myself for whatever was coming next in this bizarre, complicated case. I guessed that she would want to banish all implants from her system.

'I would like to have the left one out as well,' Amina confirmed. 'Goodness knows what would happen if I had another implant in the right side. At the moment I look totally ridiculous. I hide myself away in my office at work and rarely come out to see anyone. I go straight home, whereas I used to enjoy going for drinks or a meal after work. And I have no prospect of finding a new boyfriend, looking like this.'

'The future is a lot brighter now,' I insisted. 'When you came in here for the first time, your right breast was in a dreadful state. Now there is no more infection and we can make the correct decisions from this point onwards. I'll see what I can do about having the left implant removed by the NHS on psychological grounds. The only drawback is that special funding must be arranged and that can take six months to organise.'

Amina shook her head. I could tell that another six months in a state of limbo was not on the agenda.

'I need to have the other implant out now,' she stressed. 'I just can't wait. I'll have to go private again, hopefully to a decent clinic this time. It'll make another huge hole in my savings, but I have no other choice. I can't go back to that dodgy clinic again. Do you have any idea who might be able to help me?'

'Well, as it happens, I know a top cosmetic surgeon. He does private work, but he will be more expensive than the cut-price clinic. He'll do a really good job, so that may be the answer for you.'

'I should have paid proper money in the first place,' a rueful Amina sighed. 'Does he have a lot more qualifications than the people at the useless clinic?'

'Well, for a start, people should always check that their surgeon is registered with the General Medical Council. If you see "FRCS (Plast)" after the surgeon's name, you will know that the surgeon is a Fellow of the Royal College of Surgeons, with a special qualification in plastic surgery. That means they are skilled in carrying out all kinds of cosmetic surgery.'

I provided my friend Timothy's details, but asked Amina to research other surgeons, too. She had the choice of checking out their qualifications, looking at case studies, working out the costs involved and coming to the right decision.

She ended up choosing Timothy for the operation. After her initial consultation with him, she arrived at the surgery to see me in much better spirits. I watched her stride across the road, exuding more confidence and even helping a flustered Dr David to ease his car into a tight spot.

'Hello again, I'm back,' Amina announced as she approached the well-worn chair in front of my desk. 'Your Timothy is definitely the man, but there are still a few hurdles to cross.'

'Oh?' I asked, wondering what they could be.

'Well, he talked me through everything,' Amina explained. 'He's going to remove the left implant, but he can't do anything about my pathetic, empty right breast. I wanted to know if he could fix the scarring and the horrible stretched skin.'

'Timothy said not to touch it,' I guessed while she paused for a moment.

'Yes, he said it should be left as it is. He warned me that any further surgery would probably make matters worse. He said that, because of the extensive infection after the previous operation, it might not heal properly and end up looking worse.'

I knew that Timothy always gave spot-on advice. 'Go with what he says. If he advises leaving the right breast alone, then in my opinion that is what must happen. He's carried out countless operations like this and I have never heard of one complaint.'

Amina agreed and arranged to have the operation to remove the left implant. The breast, of course, appeared saggy and stretched after the procedure and it was a different shape to the scarred right one. Timothy did everything he could, but the previous damage inflicted was irreparable.

I hoped that Amina could start to move on with her life now, but a year after Timothy's operation, she was back in the surgery. She looked dreadful; her eyes were bloodshot; her hair was all over the place; her clothes didn't seem to fit properly; and she looked a total mess.

'I still haven't come to terms with the way I look,' she spluttered. 'I've been in here so many times, we've discussed the same things, and my life is still a disaster.'

'Would some counselling help?' I offered, hopefully. 'Perhaps we can make you less conscious of your body.'

'No thanks,' Amina said, as glum as ever. 'I just want one thing. I want to look the way I did before all this started, and that doesn't seem possible. Perhaps it is possible? Maybe I could sue the cowboys at the private clinic who caused all these problems in the first place?'

'Take legal advice,' I advised. 'You don't want to throw good money after bad.'

Amina paused for a few seconds, deep in thought. 'I know a smart lawyer who works for my insurance company. If I give him all the details he might be able to help me. That's what I'll do. I'll write everything down and see if he can give me some advice about how to get some compensation.'

Nine months passed and I didn't hear a peep. There

was no word from Amina at all. Even Naz and Dr David commented on the fact that Amina had disappeared. They were so used to seeing her in the surgery that her absence was noted by all the staff.

Then, just after the nine-month mark, I noticed a familiar name on my list for the day. Amina was due to see me in the afternoon. I asked myself: what lay in store this time? Had she come to terms with the way she looked? Had she made any progress suing the dreadful clinic? Had her lawyer been of assistance? All these questions filled my head as my door opened and Amina strode into the room. Tears spilled from her face once more. It was a familiar sight.

'Dr Leonard, I've taken up so much of your time and I am so sorry. Everything has backfired again. My lawyer wrote a letter to them and after that they offered to carry out corrective surgery on my right breast.'

'Oh?' I asked. I realised inwardly that the clinic thought it would be cheaper than a financial compensation payout. Please, please, I thought, don't tell me you went back there.

'I saw a foreign doctor and his English was poor, but he said they would make sure they made a really good job of the operation. And they would do it all for free. It seemed too good an offer to refuse. I couldn't cope with my body as it was, and there was no way I could afford to have it done privately by your man for years – even if he agreed to do it.'

'So what happened?'

'I can't believe it but it was the same old story all over again. I asked to see the exact surgeon before the operation, but no one came. I just saw some bloke with a foreign accent in the anaesthetic room, who said everything would be fine. I have no idea who he was – the surgeon or the anaesthetist. I felt like running out, but it was too late then. Next thing I knew I was in the recovery room. I have no idea who carried out the operation. I was discharged with hardly any follow-up instructions and no follow-up appointment. They tried to correct their earlier surgery, but the breast still feels terrible. Would you mind having a look?'

Back behind the familiar blue curtains, I could see that the right breast was in a real mess again. I wasn't sure what the surgeon had tried to achieve; all I could see was a fresh wound and, you've guessed, it was badly infected. I prescribed more antibiotics and Fiona applied more dressings.

'I'm not happy about this,' Dr David grumbled as he sat down for one of our early evening brainstorming sessions. 'That poor woman has had to go through all this because the cosmetics industry gets away with murder. Yes, they are getting away with murder, these people.'

Naz agreed. 'I've just had a woman in who had a nasty infected area on her upper lip. She said it was an insect bite but, looking at her, I reckon it was from a filler injection. Her upper lip was way bigger than it should have been. It looked really odd, with her lip slightly everted, bending outwards.'

'I imagine that there will be many cases like this,' I added. 'I would question the qualifications of these people, all the dubious small print, no follow-up treatment and all the other issues.'

'The whole thing stinks,' Fiona chipped in. 'I've applied all the dressings and, I can tell you, some of these clinics should be stopped now. They left Amina in a terrible state and, even when the infections set in, they weren't interested. The proper surgeon's work was a different kettle of fish but, by then, the damage had been done.'

'The stable door was closed long after the horse was halfway across the field,' Dr David added in his unique style. 'What can be done, Rosemary? You have the contacts. We don't want to see another case like that in this surgery. What can you do? How is your patient now?'

'Well, Amina has eventually agreed to have counselling,' I replied. 'But it will take a long time for her wounds to heal, in every sense. I am not sure, as a person, whether she will ever heal.'

Eventually, the wound did heal, but the scar was worse than before. Treatment-wise, we had come to the end of the road. The NHS could do no more. Two years on, Amina is scarred, emotionally as well as physically. She hates her body and hasn't had a relationship since the original operation. She is too ashamed to show her breasts to anyone.

It was partly because of Amina's case that, when asked by Professor Sir Bruce Keogh to be one of the experts advising the government on the regulation of cosmetic surgery, I readily agreed. She isn't the only tragic case I have come across. Apart from several more infected 'insect bites' on faces, I've seen lopsided eyes from Botox injections. It was a privilege to serve on the panel with Sir Bruce. The review group went into the cosmetics business in great depth and discovered that this industry, designed to make people look beautiful, had a really ugly side.

Our report questioned the competence of some 'fly in, fly out' surgeons, who were coming in from abroad. A number of these people appear to be qualified in ear, nose and throat surgery but not in plastic surgery. We could see that these surgeons, not based in the UK, were flying in and out just to earn money and gain experience at the hands of the gullible British public.

The review found that some television programmes and magazine features appeared to persuade women to have breast implants, nose jobs and injectable dermal fillers. These programmes and features made cosmetic procedures appear to be an attractive proposition, but didn't do enough to warn about the risks involved. Our panel was concerned that these fillers could be bought online, and that almost anyone could inject them in an effort to provide a youthful appearance.

The report concluded: 'It is our view that dermal fillers are a crisis waiting to happen. Dermal fillers are a particular cause for concern, as anyone can set themselves up as a practitioner with no knowledge, training or previous experience. Nor are there sufficient checks in place with regard to product quality. Most dermal fillers have no more controls than a bottle of floor cleaner.'

This sentence summed up our findings: 'A person having a non-surgical cosmetic intervention has no more protection than someone buying a ballpoint pen or a toothbrush.'

We recommended that these wrinkle-smoothing fillers should be available only on prescription. After all, they are injected beneath the skin – not a job for the amateur.

Our review also studied the aftermath of the PIP breast-implant scandal. Low-quality, industrial-grade silicone was found in implants made by the French company. We discovered that some private clinics did not even have a record of who had received the implants and, as I found with Amina, the follow-up care was atrocious.

Sir Bruce pointed out: 'At the heart of this report is the person who chooses to have a cosmetic procedure. We have heard terrible reports about people who have trusted a cosmetic practitioner to help them out but, when things have gone wrong, they have been left high and dry with no help. These people have not had the safety net which is provided by the NHS.'

We called for the banning of digitally enhanced, misleading adverts and time-limited financial incentives. We asked that an insurance scheme be put in place so that victims of failed cosmetic surgery would be able to receive compensation.

At the time of writing, the crackdown on unscrupulous clinics is underway. The Health Minister Dan Poulter said he agreed with our recommendations. He pointed out that there are responsible clinics and they do take proper care of their patients but he stressed that cowboy firms or individuals were out to make a quick profit. They did not care what happened to the people who'd been ripped off. Personally, I am aghast that hundreds of women have had to have corrective procedures on the NHS.

To Amina and countless other victims throughout the UK: this chapter is dedicated to you.

CHAPTER SEVEN

LIVING ON THE PATCH

'Where is the gold? Give me the gold now!'

My two sons were flabbergasted. 'We don't have any gold.'

'Where does your mother keep 'er jewellery?'

'She doesn't tell us where she keeps things,' twelve-year-old William answered truthfully. 'What are you going to do to us?'

'Please leave us and go away,' his brother Thomas pleaded. 'You're frightening us. What is this all about?'

We had unloaded the car on a Sunday afternoon after a few days away. I'd left the boys to unpack their bags while I nipped over to the local supermarket for milk and a few odds and ends. That was when the 'pretend' patient seized his opportunity. With me out of the way, he hobbled to our front door on a crutch. My sons are trained to look out of the front windows to see who is calling; they know not to open the door to complete strangers except under exceptional circumstances.

On this occasion, the man appeared to be genuinely injured and, therefore, my boys assumed that he was a patient needing medical help. They opened the door and, as soon as that happened, he forgot about his injured leg and charged inside.

'There must be gold in a house like this – you'd better tell me where it is NOW,' he threatened.

'We've already told you,' my sons repeated. 'There is no gold and we can't help you any more.'

Thomas, two years older than William, was cool, calm and very collected. He could tell that the aggressive rogue was an opportunist. The man, a stocky individual in his forties with a fake limp, had obviously seen me heading off to the shops. Perhaps he was new to the area; he could even have been an ex-patient from years ago with a grudge. Whatever category he fell into, this rotund intruder posed a serious threat to my family.

He was becoming more and more insistent. 'That mother of yours has jewellery. Look at your lifestyle. Of course she has gold and silver and maybe even diamonds, eh? This is your last chance. Tell me where it is and nothing will happen to you.'

Meanwhile, I sped around the supermarket, pleased to be back after our time away and looking forward to cooking supper. I loaded chicken, vegetables and a few of the boys' favourites on to the trolley as I prepared the meal in my head.

I could never have imagined, in my worst nightmares, what was happening less than a mile away – a modern-day pirate was trying to track down my non-existent gold bullion. More importantly, my sons were in danger.

Whenever we left the house I had a habit of spreading my valuables around. I have a few rings, earrings and bracelets, passed down through my family over the generations; they don't have much monetary value, but are sentimental treasures. With so many criminals looking for a pay day, I also have a small, hefty safe bolted to the floor hidden in a wardrobe. The combination that opens the door is in my head and a safe box at the bank.

'Welcome back,' Janet bellowed from the other end of the dairy produce aisle. 'Did you enjoy your escape to the West Country?'

I waved, realising that I was trapped, and steered the trolley in Janet's direction. She'd been a patient for as long as I could remember with a host of ailments from chills to bunions. Since her husband died five years ago, those conditions had increased in number. She just wanted someone to talk to. A wiry pensioner in her seventies with grey hair and the thickest glasses in South London, Janet made a beeline for me. Her trolley snaked along the aisle, neatly rounding anyone in her path. She braked, just in time to avoid a mid-aisle collision.

'It always rains in the West Country,' she informed

me. 'Do you know it always rains in the West Country?'

'Yes, I've just taken the boys down for a break with my mother in Dorset, so not all the way west. They love the sea and the walks, but it did pour down every day without fail. We still had fun and it was good to be out in the fresh air, even if we did get a bit wet . . .'

'I once had a friend in Polperro, but she died,' Janet sighed. 'I don't know anyone else down there. It's a lovely small fishing village with a quaint harbour.'

'We didn't go as far as Cornwall, but the seafood is good in Dorset,' I replied, trying not to appear rude about her geography. 'Anyway, it was nice seeing you, Janet.'

'My big toe is playing up again,' she said as she cornered me in front of the carrots. 'Would you mind having a look? The nail has come off and it is so, so painful.'

'I can't really look at it here,' I ventured, not sure if she really expected me to start examining her feet in the middle of the vegetable section. 'But, if you call up tomorrow for an appointment, I am sure we can fit you in.'

I knew I could look forward to an extensive list of ailments, including the new big toe issue, but it was all part of my working day. Anyway, I remembered in the back of my mind that Janet's blood pressure was due for a check.

As I live right in the middle of the practice area, I am

used to being approached whenever I venture out. It's rare that I manage any shopping without someone coming up to me. Generally, I love it; it's part of being in a community. The trouble is, sometimes I know who the person is and sometimes I don't. Occasionally it isn't a patient who accosts me but someone who has seen me on TV or recognised my face from articles in newspapers and magazines. This greatly amuses my sons when they are with me. They've learned to recognise the slightly quizzical look on my face when I am making small talk with a stranger.

'You didn't have a clue who that was, did you?'

'No,' would be my truthful answer.

Back in the house, the boys played for time, but the intruder was pushing for information. He was becoming more and more agitated.

Looking back now, from the details supplied by the boys, he was obviously high on drugs. His eyes bulged, he became more and more anxious, and he kept checking his inside pocket. My boys, who provided this exact account of the incident, feared that their nemesis had a knife in his pocket.

'Right, you two are going to help me,' the raider hissed menacingly. 'You say you don't know where 'er stuff is. You'll know where 'er room is, though, eh?'

The boys could hardly deny knowledge of where I slept, and so they led him upstairs to my bedroom. He sat them on one side of my bed, while on the other side he started going through the drawers in my dressing table.

At this stage my confused sons were thinking – was this guy just here for a quick smash-and-grab or was he capable of taking hostages until he got what he wanted? If he didn't get what he was looking for, would he turn violent? Were their lives in danger? The boys decided not to say that someone might arrive in the house soon, because the man's behaviour appeared to be so unpredictable.

As they sat in silence, Thomas thought to himself, 'I know this house far better than that guy. I could get out faster than him. Maybe I should leg it? If he did catch me, what would he do? Would it be any worse than what might happen if we sit here and he finds nothing? Surely he wouldn't harm William while I go for help?'

The drugged invader helped Thomas make up his mind. After a good rummage through the drawers, nothing could be found. The unwelcome visitor snarled, walked round the bed and placed his forehead a few inches from the boys. The man's eyes bulged, his breath stank of beer and he paced around the floor. He produced a roll-up machine, sat on the bed beside them and made himself a rough-looking cigarette. Goodness knows what it contained, thought Thomas.

'I'm gonna count to ten. You two are bright boys. You can count to ten with me.'

William became anxious. 'Why are you counting to ten?'

'You two have a chance to be really good boys by telling me about your mum's hiding places. You've got some idea, haven't you, boys?'

'No ideas,' Thomas shook his head.

'One. Two.'

'Not a clue,' William confirmed.

'Three.'

'What's going on?' Thomas asked, trying to hide his fear.

'Four.'

'Please stop this,' William cried. 'What have we done to deserve this?'

'Five. Six.'

'I promise you that we don't know,' Thomas said firmly. 'We honestly don't know. If we did we would tell you, just to get you out of here.'

'Seven.'

The boys looked at each other, terrified, as the uncouth intruder continued to count. He tossed some low value bracelets in his hands, obviously not satisfied with his haul so far.

'Eight.'

My son had no idea what 'nine' or 'ten' would bring; he had no intention of finding out. Thomas was off! The desperate robber was caught totally by surprise as my brave boy leaped from the bed and on to the carpet. He turned the door knob, slammed the door behind him and raced down the stairs in record time; actually he plummeted down the stairs. He could hear the robber swinging open the door and striding out of the room. The thought of that spurred Thomas on and he plunged headlong down the staircase, ending up in a crumpled heap beside the front door.

With all his remaining strength, urged on by the pounding sound of the robber on the stairs, Thomas turned the lock and virtually punched the front door open. He used every ounce of energy in his body to reach the vicarage next door and rang the ornate Victorian doorbell.

Those thirty seconds felt like an eternity as the vicar clambered down his own staircase to find out who was at the door.

'Hello, Thomas,' the friendly vicar addressed my shivering son.

'Robbery,' Thomas said at once, pointing to our house and not knowing what had happened to the robber or his brother.

I drove our estate car back from the supermarket, carrying an assortment of plastic bags filled with milk, pasta, bundles of vegetables and mounds of fruit. I thought nothing of the police sirens and speeding police cars as I drove, humming along to a song by Genesis. A helicopter overhead meant nothing to me; emergency services going about their daily business are a routine sight in South London.

Living on the Patch

I indicated to pull into our driveway and panicked as I saw two police vans parked outside. Two police vans? What the hell was going on?

I stumbled out of the car and tried to take in the scene. The vicar had his arms around both boys in the driveway, several police officers were carrying out a fingertip search, and a senior officer was talking to his headquarters, while several police radios gave out intermittent bursts of information. I recognised the names of our local streets and took in the fact that a robber – possibly armed – was on the loose.

'Dr Leonard? I'm PC Mackieson. Your sons are safe, as you can see. I'm afraid they were held in your house against their will and now a large search is under-way.'

'What happened? What happened?' I blurted out as I smothered the boys in hugs.

'The robber legged it only a short time after I legged it,' Thomas said, clearly shaken and fighting back tears, and recounting the 'hostage' story in a series of brief instalments.

'The man certainly has legged it,' the policeman added. 'We were just about to go inside the house when William appeared at the door. By that time the robber obviously knew the game was up and had disappeared.'

William, of course, had no idea where the intruder had gone; he didn't know Thomas's whereabouts; and he'd been understandably reluctant to open the door

147

again. However, the welcome racket outside caused by the police prompted him to turn the lock.

Both boys gave lengthy statements to the police to help in their search. Would the intruder strike somewhere else? We had no knowledge of his background or movements. Despite a city-wide police search, our pathetic robber was never caught. All he received for his efforts were several pairs of low-value earrings and bracelets.

Victim Support played a crucial role in talking to my boys after their frightening experience. I resented the fact that my sons had been put through this ordeal and very much welcomed Victim Support's comforting approach. Ten years on both boys, now young men, still remember the incident clearly; they always go through a rigorous checking process before they open the door to anyone.

Sometimes, though, that door is right to be opened . . .

As my house is only half a mile from the surgery and I live among my patients, there is no point in trying to hide. In fact, my patients are usually very protective of me.

My back garden, containing my precious vegetable patch, is overlooked by a block of flats. These can only be bought by people who are over fifty-five years old. The residents keep an eye on my house, although I have never asked them to do so. They are vigilant when I am on holiday or during the day when I'm working in the surgery. That vile intruder would have been reported in seconds had he chosen the back of the house to make his entrance.

A few weeks after the hostage drama, and with the entire street on alert, I arrived home after a long day in the surgery. I could tell that something was wrong when I pulled up in the driveway. Jessie, one of the residents from the flats, was standing by the side gate.

'Some kids climbed over your back wall,' Jessie yelled. 'A few of them were running around your garden.'

'Did they take anything?' I asked.

'One of them took a cucumber and he was about to uproot your potatoes.'

I was intrigued. 'What happened next?'

'I put on my slippers and chased them around the garden and out along the street. It's the least I could do after you prescribed those painkillers for my lumbago. Those kids won't be back.'

Jessie, still fairly fit in her eighties, was typical of those loyal residents in the block of flats. I grinned at the thought of her racing along the street in her pink fluffy slippers, chasing the boys and the cucumber. I decided that I could afford to lose the cucumber, but I did think that the youngsters probably had something more valuable in mind when they climbed over the wall.

Inevitably, many of the patients who live locally are also my friends. Like all doctors, everything that is said to me in my professional capacity is absolutely confidential, and I've never had a problem with combining the roles of doctor and friend. In most rural communities this is the norm; the local doctor is part of the community and always has been.

When you have to do visits late into the evening and sometimes at night, it makes sense to live close to your patients. Increasingly, though, especially in towns and cities, GPs no longer do night work and so they actively avoid living near to their patients; they prefer to separate work and leisure. I am one of the exceptions.

'Another glass of wine, Amanda?' I offered as my friend took the final sip from her glass of Chablis – half price at the local off-licence.

I had decided to try something different from my weekday favourite Pinot Grigio. I love top-quality vino on a special occasion and I had splashed out on a case of the Chablis as I was hosting a dinner party for my oldest friend, who was celebrating fifty years on the planet. My research on fine wine told me that I should try this Vielles Vignes, or 'old vines', with my chicken in white wine sauce. I used a cheaper wine to make the dish, though! The online review said that my chosen wine for the evening was produced from forty-year-old vines in the heart of the Chablis region. I liked the idea of traditional methods and a long ageing process. The long ageing process hadn't taken its toll on Amanda, though, who did not look remotely as if she had reached her half century.

Living on the Patch

The guest list featured Amanda and her husband, plus a cross section of friends, many of whom were also patients. I was pleased that they all enjoyed the main course – I'd served it with loads of vegetables and I was delighted to announce that many of the ingredients had come from my back garden.

As I poured some more of the chilled Chablis into Amanda's glass, I could hear a knock on the front door. Who could that be? A robber? A cucumber thief? Could it be William, returning to the house instead of having his sleepover at Mark's?

'Best not to answer it,' Amanda advised as her husband, Rob, nodded. 'Remember what happened last time.'

'I have a spy hole now,' I replied. 'If I don't know who it is, I won't answer it.'

I could see through the spy hole that it was my friend Maggie standing there with her fourteen-year-old son. Glass in hand, I opened the door. 'What happened, Maggie? Is Sean OK?' Although I could see that he was far from OK.

His mum filled me in on the details. 'He was riding his bike along our street and, for some reason, collided with the kerb. He managed to get himself home, dripping with blood, and when I'd cleaned him up I could see he had a large graze on his knee. But I'm more worried about that gash on his chin.'

I was also worried about the gash on his chin. Sean

was a close friend of William and, like my son, he didn't make a fuss over nothing. It was unusual for him to be close to tears. His wound needed immediate attention.

'Come in, come in,' I insisted as the two of them huddled in the porch. I could see that they were embarrassed to come over on a Saturday evening; but Maggie, living two streets away, had chosen the quickest and easiest option to get help for her son.

I ushered the pair into our lounge, which was tidier than usual because of the invited guests. I'd planned to serve coffee there and so an assortment of candles greeted mother and son as they walked in and sat down. I thought briefly about the blood on the cream sofa covers. Too bad, I thought. People come first.

I hastily grabbed some tissues. 'That cut is about two inches long and it's quite deep,' I told Maggie as I applied pressure and kept the flow of blood to a minimum, for Sean's sake as well as the sofa covers. 'It's bleeding quite heavily so it really needs urgent treatment.'

As is the case with many doctors, the first aid kit in my house isn't a small box; it's more a cupboard full of pills, creams and different dressings. I keep a supply of Steri-strips, which are thin, adhesive strips for use in closing small wounds, and a recent, very useful addition to my medical store is surgical glue for pulling together small cuts. I also keep a suture kit, which is ideal for stitching wounds in an emergency. This is kept with some local anaesthetic, although thankfully I have rarely had to use it.

Living on the Patch

The knee needed a good scrub to remove the dirt, but the chin needed suturing. In a less obvious place it would have been possible to glue it, and then hold the wound with Steri-strips. But on a patient's face a good cosmetic result is important, and that can only be achieved with sutures.

I studied the gash again, stemmed the flow of blood, and voiced my concerns to Maggie. I was worried about working on Sean's face; a bad cut could show up as a scar. 'Maggie, I think he should go to A and E. That cut needs stitches. I've had a glass of wine and it's important to get everything done correctly.'

'Rosemary, please,' Maggie pleaded. 'A and E on a Saturday night? We'll never get seen. Even if we do get treated tonight, how do I know who would do the stitching? Please can't you do it?'

I understood her fears about the local A and E on a Saturday night. Even on weekdays it was extremely busy. On Saturdays there was the additional workload caused by people who'd had too much to drink and the fights and brawls, often involving broken bottles, that then ensued. Plus, staff had to deal with the occasional stabbing. Despite the best efforts of the fabulous, hardworking staff, I'd heard from patients that waits of several hours were quite common. It certainly wouldn't be my first choice of where to spend a Saturday evening!

'Yes, I could deal with Sean,' I admitted, 'but the wound is on his face. It really needs to be done carefully and, apart from anything else, I've had a glass of wine.'

Maggie pleaded again, 'I'd rather that you did it, even after a glass of wine.'

I continued to stem the flow of blood and pondered over my next move.

'You're not drunk, Rosemary,' Maggie continued. 'In fact, you are not even remotely slurring your words. Surely you can do it here? You know Sean is the same as William – they love all sports. You know how much they enjoy rugby, skiing and mountain biking. This isn't his first injury and it won't be his last. If he does end up with a small scar on his chin, so be it. What do you think, Sean?'

'The last friend of mine who went to A and E was there for six hours and I'm not planning to be a male model,' he answered. 'A small scar isn't important. It might even make me look more macho. Why would I worry?'

I left mother and son on the sofa while I returned to the dining room. 'A small emergency,' I announced and explained what had happened. 'Maggie has asked me to do the stitching, but I'm worried because I've been drinking. How much have I had? Am I in a fit state to be doing suturing? Tell me honestly.'

'You've been busy cooking and, as far as I remember, you've not had very much at all,' Rob confirmed. 'You've only had one small glass . . . for a change,' he added mischievously.

I still wasn't sure about taking the job on. I took a lot of persuading. The dinner guests all had their say, but they agreed that A and E on a Saturday night was worth avoiding, if possible. They confirmed that I did not appear at all drunk and that I seemed fit to do the stitching.

'I bet some doctors at the hospital are working after a beer or two,' Amanda added. 'It's just that no one knows.'

Even so, I thought, it wasn't good for their patients. I returned to the lounge.

Maggie looked at me pleadingly, 'Please say you're not going to send us to A and E for such a little thing . . .'

'OK, I'll do it. Obviously there are risks associated with carrying out a procedure at home, so you will have to sign a consent form. I haven't got any here, so I'll have to handwrite it. Is that OK? I've just got to cover myself . . .'

'I'll sign anything. Just give me the form and I'll sign it.'

I was aware that several witnesses knew that I had explained all the risks. However, I also knew that suturing with wine on board, in my home, was not exactly best medical practice. But it crossed my mind that, once they got home and contemplated spending the night at A and E, patching up the wound until the following morning might seem like a good idea, but that wasn't ideal, either.

The kitchen was cluttered with the preparations for dinner, so we decided the best place for the stitching was my bathroom. First I had to locate the suturing kit, and cursed the fact I hadn't tidied up my medical cupboard in the utility room. I eventually found a sterile syringe, needle, a vial of local anaesthetic, and also the suture and the sterile instruments required for the delicate procedure.

'Could you sit on the loo, Sean?' I asked my unexpected patient as I continued to stem the flow of blood. 'Just sit very still and we can get this done quickly.'

'I like the sound of that,' his mother said. 'I will never be able to thank you enough for this. I'm also aware that we've broken up your dinner party.'

'Don't worry, we will continue with that in a few moments. I'm keen to get this wound treated.'

Ever so gently, I infiltrated the wound with local anaesthetic. I waited for a couple of minutes until the area was numb and then sutured it up.

'There you go,' I proclaimed proudly as I admired my work. 'It's stopped bleeding now.'

'Those stitches are really neat,' Maggie complimented me. 'How did you make them so neat? You must be an expert at sewing trousers!'

'It's probably the wine,' I joked. 'Perhaps it helped me concentrate and produce good stitching work. I wouldn't normally recommend wine before doing this, though!'

Sean was thrilled. 'I can spend the rest of the night at

home, playing computer games, instead of sitting around at the hospital.'

'Please don't tell anyone that I am carrying out emergency repairs on Saturday evenings, especially on the loo!' I warned him with a smile. 'I'm not even going to tell Fiona, my practice nurse, as she would tell me off. By the way, where's your mum?' While talking to Sean and scrutinising my work in the loo, I hadn't noticed Maggie leave. I'd replied to her comment about the stitches, but hadn't seen her since.

'I don't know. She was outside your loo door a few minutes ago.'

The doorbell rang. Who on earth could that be? Had someone else fallen off a bike? Was it a car crash victim? Had Jessie tripped over while checking on my vegetable patch? Would I ever get down to enjoying Amanda's birthday party?

I bounded down the stairs, prepared for yet another emergency – or perhaps William's return – and could see a woman through the spy hole. Maggie was standing there, beaming from ear to ear. I opened the door.

'Here you are,' Maggie grinned. 'Enjoy the rest of your evening.'

Maggie had managed to fit in a speedy visit to the off-licence down the road. She handed me a bottle in a presentation box, while the newly repaired Sean appeared from the loo and joined his mother on the doorstep. I tried hard to refuse her offering, but to no avail.

I hugged Maggie and Sean and headed back to the dining room where copious amounts of my prized Chablis were being consumed.

'Could someone pour me a glass of this?' I asked with a sense of urgency in my voice, at the same time showing off my gift for the evening's work.

Rob unwrapped the box, prepared the opener with a flourish, and looked at the label. 'There must be a good offer at the off-licence,' he said. 'Look – more Chablis!'

I took a decent gulp, joined in the laughter and scampered off to the kitchen to prepare the dessert – a trifle, with not a trace of alcohol!

CHAPTER EIGHT

A MATTER OF TASTE

I was doctor turned detective again when Georgie came to see me. I had solved some tricky cases in my time but, with Georgie, the evidence was flimsy and confusing, witnesses were few and far between, there were no similar incidents to give me ideas, and basically I was stumped.

Georgie was a pretty young woman aged around twenty-four. I could tell she had been well brought up. She spoke with a 'proper' accent, far removed from the day-to-day South London dialect I usually came across. I remembered her from several years ago and recalled that she had attended a local private school. I used to be on nodding terms with her parents, although I hadn't seen them for a long time.

Now Georgie sat opposite me, dressed in modern Sloane attire – skinny jeans, ballet pumps, a tight jumper and the shortest of short jackets. I thought she looked a bit thin. It could be that she was a natural 'skinny', I concluded, but I wondered whether she was eating healthily.

'How is life treating you?' I enquired, noting that her entire demeanour oozed success. 'The last I heard you were entering the world of public relations.'

'That's correct,' Georgie answered in well-rehearsed clipped tones. 'I'm organising all sorts of events from garden parties to corporate lunches. I write all the press releases and sort everything out, basically.'

'It's great to see you moving up in the world,' I smiled. 'What brings you here today? Is it a general check-up? I haven't seen you for a few years.'

Georgie's expression changed in an instant. 'Well, it's all very embarrassing, Dr Rosemary. I'm not sure what is going on with my body. I just need someone to talk to and perhaps make some suggestions.'

'Well, there is no need to be embarrassed,' I assured her. 'I deal with all sorts of people with embarrassing problems. It's just part of my job. What can I do to help?'

'Well, I have itchy nipples. I'm worried about it. My friend said it was because I was coming to the end of my period. She even said I might be pregnant. But I had another thought: could it be breast cancer? I know people who've died from breast cancer.'

'Hold on a minute,' I said before she could continue with her list of possible causes. 'First of all, when was your last period?'

'A couple of weeks ago.'

'And was it normal?'

'Yes, just a few days, as always.'

'And what are you doing for contraception?'

'I'm on the pill and I haven't missed any.'

I reassured her that, from what she had said, she was most unlikely to be pregnant. Even if she was pregnant, it tended to cause sore, rather than itchy, nipples.

'So what about breast cancer?' She looked at me anxiously.

'I'm glad you've come to see me because your friend is putting so many false ideas in your head. For a start, both your nipples are itchy. Almost always, breast cancer symptoms appear in one breast at a time and hardly ever cause itchy nipples. But I'll examine you, of course, to put your mind at rest.'

I chatted to her while she undressed and established that there were no other breast symptoms, no nipple discharge and no itching anywhere else. The most common reason I see for this is usually a seam in a bra causing irritation, especially if the bra is made from lace. But she was wearing a smooth-cupped bra and said she hardly ever wore anything else. 'It gives a better line under my clothes.'

I had a good look at her nipples. They were, indeed, dry and cracked. Then I checked her breasts for lumps and, as I expected, her breast tissue felt completely normal.

161

'Well, Georgie, it looks like eczema. I'm certain that it is nothing serious.'

Georgie looked relieved. 'Eczema? I haven't had anything like that before. Why is it affecting my nipples?'

'Well, it is also called dermatitis and, just in one place, it's usually a sign that something is irritating your skin. The most common reason I see for breast eczema, apart from scratchy, lacy bras, is biological detergents, or perfumed fabric conditioners. It's true that there's a rare form of breast cancer that can cause an itchy, red rash on the nipple, but your nipples don't have that appearance. Anyway, it only affects one nipple and not both at the same time.'

'I'm not sure what my bras are washed in,' she admitted. 'I share my flat with three other people and we just buy a huge box of whatever is cheapest at the supermarket.'

'Check the label. It will say if it is non-biological,' I advised. 'And avoid using perfumed soaps, shower gels, bath oils and the like. Try to use products with no added perfumes and ensure that they are suitable for sensitive skin.'

'OK, I'll try,' she agreed.

I prescribed that old favourite, hydrocortisone ointment, to be used twice a day. I also needed to keep tabs on her because of the very slight chance of an underlying breast problem.

'Please follow all that advice, use the cream and come back if there is no improvement.'

A month later, Lizzy buzzed through, 'That lady Georgie would like to make an appointment. She's keen to see you tomorrow. You've a spare telephone appointment slot – could I fit her in for that?'

'Yes, that will be OK,' I replied. We had recently started providing bookable telephone appointments, for problems that can be discussed over the phone, to save both the doctor's and patient's time. Many of my patients are now monitoring their own blood pressure at home and often they just need to call me to discuss the result.

I called Georgie on her mobile but it soon became clear that I needed to see her breasts again in the surgery.

Instead of her previous, confident stride and management-style demeanour, she ambled across the floor with her head down; she looked totally down in the dumps. Detective Leonard was called upon yet again.

'It's like I said on the phone,' she explained. 'My nipples did get better but they've flared up again. Not only that, I have strange patches on my tummy. What is going on, Dr Rosemary?'

In the familiar surroundings of my examination couch, I could tell that all was not well. Her nipples were cracked and sore again, and I could see patches of eczema on her tummy. But what was the cause? Eczema is a common enough problem, especially in South

London where the hard water appears to be very skin-unfriendly.

'We're going to sort this out,' I promised. 'Could you tell me what you are using to wash your clothes, and your body?'

Georgie had tried her best to comply with my suggestions. 'I'm using non-biological washing powders for sensitive skin. I've taken your advice on soap, shower gel and everything else. I go through a daily routine of double checking everything and then I turn up here looking like the pits.'

'It's not great,' I agreed. 'I'll prescribe more hydrocortisone ointment. With eczema, prevention is better than cure, though. Make sure you use plenty of moisturisers to stop your skin becoming dry – twice a day, morning and evening. That's often an underlying problem in skin when it is prone to eczema.'

Was the case solved? Another month passed and Georgie was sitting in the chair opposite me once more. She'd followed my guidelines, covered herself in moisturisers regularly and used the hydrocortisone ointment every day. We trooped back behind the curtains around my couch once more.

This time, I could see several patches of really inflamed skin on her stomach. The skin on her breasts was red; it was inflamed and weeping in places. It looked as though the patches of eczema had become infected. This can happen when the organisms that normally live on the skin start multiplying in the inflamed areas. They produce toxins which then cause further inflammation, creating a very nasty experience for the patient. There is infection, inflammation, more infection, even more inflammations, and a totally unpleasant life for the sufferer.

Georgie's face had a glum, downcast expression. 'I appreciate everything you're doing, Dr Rosemary, but I'm not improving at all. I'm taking up hours of your time – and we're getting nowhere.'

'Don't get disheartened,' I said encouragingly. 'We will find out what is causing this.'

'What else do you suggest?' Georgie asked.

'Eczema can be triggered by house dust mites,' I pointed out. 'Do you have any old furnishings, mattresses or carpets in your flat? The only way we can solve this is to go through every potential cause.'

'All my stuff is fairly new. I do have an old teddy bear on top of a dusty wardrobe, but that's all that I can think of. Could my bear be to blame? I've had her for more than twenty years without any problems.'

I liked the fact she'd referred to her bear as a female. My old teddy bear is a girl, too, and still lives in a corner of my bedroom. 'Put her in your freezer for twenty-four hours to kill off any mites,' I suggested hopefully. 'After that, run a vacuum cleaner over her to remove any remaining dust. Is she dressed, like mine?'

'Yes, she is dressed.'

'Well, wash the clothes, too – at sixty degrees if that's possible without wrecking them – to kill off any mites lingering there. Plus, give your house a thorough clean, including the top of that wardrobe, and we'll take things from there.'

A smiling Georgie returned to the surgery a couple of weeks later with much-improved skin. I couldn't conceal my joy, wished Georgie well and waved as she left. What a result, I thought, and then wondered whether I should give my bear similar treatment. My son William had eczema and, though we'd thoroughly cleaned his room and old soft toys, there were several decades of dust – and probably mites – on my old bear.

A month later, though, a tearful Georgie returned to the surgery. It hadn't been a successful result after all. My hopes were shattered. All that treatment and all those conversations had been in vain.

'Doctor, this is really getting me down,' she wept. 'Look at me. Look at me.'

Behind the curtain I really felt sorry for this young woman. Her condition was worse than ever with large areas of sore, weeping eczematous skin. Her breasts, as always, were worst affected, especially around her nipples, but this time she also had a red rash surrounding her pubic area.

My first thought was that her washing powder must be to blame; the rash looked angriest where her underwear had been touching her skin. But it was odd that her back was completely clear.

I suddenly had a brainwave. 'Do you use a lubricant during sex?' I asked, studying the unpleasant-looking rash around her vagina.

'Well, I don't use any lubricant but my boyfriend sometime uses chocolate fudge sauce,' she replied sheepishly.

'Sorry? What did you say? Chocolate fudge sauce?'

'Yes, he loves smothering me with different sauces and then licking them off. He's tried so many flavours. I did notice the other day that the rash appeared after he'd applied the chocolate fudge sauce. But it couldn't be that, surely?'

'Yes, I think it probably is,' I declared, trying hard not to show my surprise. 'Are these the sauces you can buy to go on ice cream?'

'Yes, and we've tried lemon sauce, chocolate sauce, cream sauce, raspberry sauce and strawberry sauce. He even uses—'

I interrupted her as this detective doctor felt that the case was almost certainly solved. 'So, Georgie, it appears there is a link with the chocolate sauce?'

Georgie continued with her saucy tale, 'Yes, thinking about it, he only uses the chocolate fudge sauce occasionally and that is when I come in to see you with all my sore bits and rashes. What's in the sauce, then, to make me flare up?'

'Without studying the ingredients, it's hard to say, but it must contain something that sets off a reaction. Goodness knows what it is. Let's face it – the stuff isn't designed to be spread all over your body and then licked off. Remember, there is a high sugar content in it, too, which is an ideal breeding-ground for bacteria. Once the skin is broken, if you put any sweet sauce on, it is more likely to get infected. You have sensitive skin, so it might be best to avoid any sauces in the future.'

Just as a formality, I invited Georgie back for a check-up a month later. What a difference a month makes. Her skin was clear, her healthy complexion caught my eye and she simply glowed with happiness.

'Sauce is off the menu?' I enquired, as tactfully as possible.

'Oh yes,' Georgie laughed. 'I threw away the chocolate fudge sauce – so that is no longer an issue.'

'I wouldn't recommend any flavour, chocolate or otherwise,' I answered, thrilled that the case had been solved.

'I have a new boyfriend,' Georgie beamed. 'And guess what?'

'He's tall, dark and handsome?'

'Wrong. He's short, blond and fairly handsome. Main thing is – he hates chocolate fudge sauce!'

I have to admit that I chortled to myself about the chocolate fudge sauce for a few days. I brought up the case at the next monthly meeting, trying hard to keep a straight face and putting forward the facts in a professional manner: Dr David said the case had broadened his horizons; Naz thought it was hysterical; and Fiona refused to believe a word.

Only a few days later, I was far from a picture of health myself. I had a cold, my nose was running and my sinuses were blocked. I always avoid being off sick if at all possible; I wasn't ill enough to stay away, but I felt very much under the weather.

I grimaced as I prepared my desk for the Monday morning surgery and checked my appointments for the day. What a collection. My list included Joe, to check on his general health and drinking habits; Edgar, an elderly man in a wheelchair who wanted to walk again; Martin, a bakery worker with a persistent cough; and Gail, a single mum in her thirties who suffered from migraines.

I checked Joe's file to ensure that his drinking was indeed on a downward spiral. Joe's last visit had proved to be a positive one with the reappearance of a vital part of his anatomy, thanks to the loss of weight. I made a mental note to check that he was persisting with two alcohol-free days a week.

I spotted one unfamiliar name on my list. The notes said that Marcia had moved to London from the north of England and needed to see a doctor as soon as possible. Doreen had fitted her in as my first patient at eight o'clock.

Doctor's Notes

At eight o'clock sharp, Marcia jogged into my consulting room. She had obviously just been to the gym and appeared in front of me wearing a sweatshirt, shorts and trainers. Her face was still sweating and her clothing had large, dark, wet patches from her exertions. Much as I encourage my patients to take physical exercise, I often wish they would return home for a shower and change before coming into the surgery – particularly if they need to be examined.

I could tell that Marcia was a fit woman. She was in her mid-thirties, perhaps, with a trim figure and had the look of a woman who worked out regularly. There was more fat on a greasy chip, as they say around these parts. I could see from Marcia's muscular arms that she made full use of the gym.

She came straight out with it, 'My boyfriend says I taste funny.' I hoped that I wasn't facing another sauce-related case. On the positive side, my recent experience had prepared me for all eventualities. 'I'm new to the area and I don't have any friends yet. I don't know what to tell my boyfriend and I can't really tell my parents. It's not really the type of thing I can discuss with them.'

'Yes, it's not a conversation to have with your parents,' I agreed.

'They have been so strict with me over the years, you know. They settled in Carlisle after coming here from the West Indies. They have a small shop up there, but it wasn't my scene. Also, it rained all the time. You know, that wind blows in from the Solway Firth and it howls along the streets.'

After Marcia's brief background chat and a Carlisle history lesson, I moved the conversation back to her 'funny taste' problem.

'You said that you taste funny? Which part of your body tastes funny? Is it your lips or your mouth?'

'No, they are OK. It's my fanny.'

'Oh, I see. It's your vagina.'

Marcia appeared more relaxed with that sensitive information out of the way. 'I moved here about two months ago and met a sensational West Indian guy. He's really good to me, you know, but he maintains that I taste funny.'

'Can you remember anyone else saying that you tasted funny? Is your boyfriend new to oral sex?'

'No, I am sure he's quite experienced. He just says I taste different. His big thing is oral sex and I have to say that it is his speciality. He's so good at it.'

I wondered what details were coming next and how I could make sure the conversation concentrated on the medical facts. 'Does this happen after you've eaten a curry, perhaps?' I suggested. 'Or could it even be something like asparagus? That can cause odd-smelling urine in some people.'

'No, it doesn't seem to happen after strong food or anything like that.'

Doctor's Notes

I asked if she had a discharge, which would be a tell-tale sign that an infection might be to blame.

'No discharge. Nothing sore down there at all.'

'How long has this been going on for?'

'It's been happening for a while now. I know that I should have come to see you ages ago but it's so embarrassing. And, anyway, it only happens occasionally. I've been doing some research on the Internet but it hasn't been much help, especially as I don't want to end up looking at a load of porn sites. The receptionist said you were the expert in women's matters, but it isn't that easy to get an appointment with you.'

It was a familiar complaint. I reckon I could work seven days a week and patients would still complain that they couldn't get in to see me. But, all the same, I apologised and said that the surgery was looking at ways of making more appointments available, which was true.

I turned my attention back to the taste issue. I kept to my normal pattern of eliminating possibility after possibility and, hopefully, homing in on the exact cause of Marcia's unfortunate problem down below.

'Has your boyfriend explained what he means by "funny"? Does he mean "fishy"? An imbalance of the natural bacteria in the vagina is called bacterial vaginosis. It's known to cause a fishy-smelling discharge.'

'He just described it as funny or odd,' Marcia said in her Cumbrian accent, with shades of Jamaican darting in and out. 'He's said this from the very start of our relationship. Could you check it out?'

The well-worn curtains were pulled across once more and my funny-tasting patient climbed on to the couch. I had to admit to myself that she did have a slight body odour, but it was of sweat. Nothing unusual about that but I wondered if that was to blame.

'Does he comment about the taste after you've been to the gym?'

'Sometimes, but I always shower when I get home. Sorry I haven't had time to do that today. But I really don't think it's linked with any exercise sessions. It seems, well, sort of random.'

'Let's have a look and see if I can find the reason,' I suggested, as I prepared a speculum, together with some swabs to check for an infection.

'Does everything look normal?' Marcia asked as I examined her.

My blocked nose meant any smell would have had to be quite strong for me to detect it. Bearing in mind her sweaty state, I was quite glad I had a cold! There was no sign of an infection and I reassured her that it all looked normal, but said I had taken swabs to check there wasn't an infection.

'Are you sure it's all normal? You have checked really carefully, haven't you?'

Surely she didn't want me to do a taste test?

I paused. 'Yes, I've done everything. This is a difficult

one to solve,' I told Marcia when she sat down in the chair again. 'Everything seems to be completely OK. Are you sure that your boyfriend isn't just having a problem with his taste buds?'

'No. He's serious about all of this and I believe it will cause us real problems soon. I can tell that he is starting to go off me because of this. There must be an answer . . .'

I sent off the swabs and, as expected, they came back as clear as a bell.

'I'm running out of ideas here,' I confessed as I phoned Marcia with the results. 'Everything is fine with no abnormalities. I'm still wondering if the problem lies with your boyfriend.'

'Could you see us together?' Marcia asked hopefully. 'Then we could sort this out once and for all.'

The suggested appearance of Marcia and her man wasn't possible. 'I can't do that as he isn't registered at my practice. Have you thought about going to a genito-urinary clinic? They might be able to find something. They have all the latest testing equipment.'

'You must be joking,' Marcia muttered, displaying a prejudiced view. 'Those places are for gays and pro-stitutes. I'm not going to sit in a waiting room with prostitutes! Can you imagine me in there with that lot, strutting their stuff all over the place? I'm not going there – no way.'

I tried to convince her that this wasn't the case, but

she was having none of it. She wanted me to deal with the problem in the surgery, where no one could have an inkling of what was wrong.

The day before Marcia's next appointment, I had a good search on the Internet. That didn't help. Many people are reluctant to admit that they have oral sex and I couldn't find any new information. There were plenty of medical sites with details about conditions and how to treat them. But because of the nature of my job, I could have written the articles myself!

However, as soon as Marcia lay on the couch during her next visit, I noticed a familiar smell around her genital area. It was such a powerful aroma. I could smell disinfectant! Detective Leonard knew that the case had been solved. 'Please get dressed and come and sit down,' I beckoned, failing to conceal my glee.

'You've found something!'

'Yes, I've smelled something. And that something smelled suspiciously like a well-known brand of disinfectant. I have a good idea what is happening here.'

'Oh, I had a bath this morning and I always put Dettol in the water.'

I beamed triumphantly. 'Dettol is a very fine product but not for your bath water. Like all disinfectants it kills off the good bacteria as well as the bad. There are good bacteria living in the vagina and when they are killed off you are at a high risk of getting an infection. Actually, you're lucky not to have one.'

'Killed off? What's that about good bacteria?' Marcia asked with a puzzled expression. 'How can I have good bacteria? I'm glad that I decided not to become a doctor. You have to know too much!'

'It is a fact that the vagina contains good and bad bacteria. The good bacteria protect against infection. Women also have a smaller amount of bad bacteria. If the bad germs outnumber the good ones, you can develop all sorts of problems. The most common one is bacterial vaginosis, which causes a fishy smell, but over-cleaning can cause thrush, too. I suspect that odd taste your boyfriend has detected is because you have an imbalance of bacteria in your vagina.'

'That does all make sense,' Marcia murmured gently, stroking her chin.

'No more disinfectant in the bath, then!'

'That will change the way we've been doing things for generations, then. My mother made me put it in my bath water, and my grandmother made her. I'm sure that it is a tradition going way back in our family. I was told it was the only way to be sure I was "clean". If anything, since this problem started, I've been using it even more.'

I nodded in agreement, 'I have heard about using disinfectant in bath water. It's mainly done by descendants of immigrants from the West Indies, which explains your family's habits. Fortunately you had a bath this morning and I knew what was happening at once.'

A Matter of Taste

'He won't want to lick me at all now, though,' Marcia groaned. 'He insists that it has to be really clean down there. This sounds bizarre. The smell will go, but my boyfriend will feel that I am not clean because I'm not using disinfectant. How daft is that!'

'He will be happy enough,' I said, confidently. 'I mean, he has been complaining about the strange taste – and that will go now. You will be surprised; I can assure you of that. Just use water. Also, the vagina cleans itself! Please explain to your boyfriend that disinfectant in bath water is not a good plan and that it's been the cause of all your problems.'

We chatted for another few minutes, breaking down a few cultural barriers and talking a lot of common sense. She came round to my way of thinking and promised to give all the details to her boyfriend, who happened to be a teacher at one of the local schools.

I saw Marcia out of the door and into reception, at the same time catching a glimpse of Fiona bustling backwards and forwards to her treatment room. I couldn't help noticing a well-known brand of disinfectant on one of the shelves.

Fiona saw me staring at the bottle. 'Do you need some disinfectant?' my practice nurse offered. 'I've got plenty of the stuff in here. I need a clear-out. I've got about seven half-used bottles. Here you are.'

'No, I'm OK,' I laughed. 'I need a break from disinfectant, if the truth be told.'

Doctor's Notes

'Dr Leonard, have you been solving more cases involving mysterious substances?'

'Yes I have,' I confirmed. 'Let's just say it was a matter of taste.'

CHAPTER NINE

WHO DO YOU
THINK I AM?

'I'm having a baby,' Samantha announced, without a trace of emotion, as she opened my door and strode across the consulting room.

'Oh great,' I answered. 'What a lovely surprise. You must be thrilled and looking forward to having your second child. It's wonderful news, isn't it?'

'No, it's not,' Samantha frowned.

'Oh?'

'It may not be my husband's baby.'

'I see,' I whispered softly, waiting for the rest of the details to emerge.

'Patrick knows I've been having an affair and now I'm pregnant, he's wondering who the father is.'

Detective Leonard realised that the investigation here

was mostly out of her hands; nature would take its course. The baby would arrive to the delight or sadness of the parents. At the moment there was confusion all around.

'Do you have a good idea who the father is?'

'I'm not sure,' Samantha said slowly, weighing up the possibilities.

With only two options available, I pressed for more information, 'Who, do you think, is more likely to be the father?'

Samantha admitted that it was a fifty–fifty situation. 'I've been so stupid. I was sleeping with Patrick and Kamran at the same time.'

'Kamran?' I ventured carefully, not knowing how much Samantha was prepared to tell me. I was happy to hear the whole story, if she would let me.

The future mum, at about seven weeks pregnant, decided to hide nothing. 'You know that my husband, Patrick, is a builder. Well, with the recession, he had to find work in the Midlands, which meant that he was away a lot during the week. I met Kamran at the gym, we chatted, and one thing led to another.'

'I can see what it led to,' I nodded.

'Patrick and I have been married for about ten years now and things have been getting stale. Kamran is young, athletic and exciting. I know that I've done something terrible and goodness knows what lies around the corner. If things go badly, Patrick will divorce me and I'll have to bring up the child on my own.'

Who Do You Think I Am?

'Kamran's younger than you?'

'I'll be thirty-five this year and he is five years younger. His parents are Pakistani, although he was born here and so he's English through and through, really.'

I studied Samantha as she talked. I'd known the family for a long time and this dreaded scenario came as a shock to me. I suppose you could say that Samantha had a 'girlie' look about her. A crueller word might be 'tarty'. She was slender and liked to show off her legs. In fact, her skirt was so short it looked more like a miniature curtain pelmet and she had to pull it down occasionally to display any sign of fabric at the tops of her legs. It seemed obvious to me that Samantha would attract interest at the gym.

I was keen to establish what I could do to help. 'How did your husband know what was going on?'

'Patrick used to be a member of the gym, too,' Samantha explained. 'He just appeared at weekends but I go there three or four times a week. My sister looks after Abbey, who's coming up for twelve now. I've had plenty of free time to go to the gym.'

'Was there no hard evidence?' I asked, hopefully.

'Unfortunately there was. Patrick saw a text appear on my phone while I was in the loo. It was a Saturday night and I should have been more careful with the phone. The message said something about looking forward to our next date. Bloody mobile phones. I was caught red-handed.'

Doctor's Notes

This wasn't the first time I'd heard about text messages revealing clandestine affairs. As Samantha sat before me facing such a predicament I thought: if you decide to play around, mobile phones are like a ticking time bomb!

'I feel such a twit,' she admitted. 'I always thought you could have sex during your period or just after and not get pregnant. Why did it all go so wrong? I even read up about safe times to have sex.'

'You'll be surprised to know that you can get pregnant at any time during your menstrual cycle. There are periods when you are most fertile, of course. The egg is released from your ovaries about twelve to fourteen days before your next period starts and that is when you are most likely to get pregnant. But, if you ovulate early, then you can get pregnant at the end of your period, or just after.'

'But when I had sex it was nowhere near that time,' Samantha groaned.

I explained that everything did not always go to plan when people used guesswork as birth control. 'Sperm can live in the body for up to seven days after sex. So you can see that there is a risk, especially if you ovulate early. The only foolproof method is proper contraception.'

'I can see it's no use crying over spilt milk,' she mused. 'Whatever was spilt, I have to keep going and live through the consequences.'

It was time to find out how her relationship was

coping with all this stress. 'Patrick is still with you, though? Do you think that the two of you can get through this, whatever the outcome? Have you thought about having a termination?'

'I did think about having an abortion and I probably should have just gone ahead and quickly got rid of the baby before anyone else knew. But Patrick won't hear of it. He can't bear the thought of getting rid of his child. I know this is all my fault and now I've just got to see it through. Being pregnant under all this pressure won't help me or the new baby. I've known you for a long time and I'm just wondering if you could give me some extra support. I don't really want to talk to anyone else.'

'What is Patrick saying?' I asked, realising that the situation was likely to deteriorate even further over the next few weeks.

'Things are really bad at home.'

'How bad?'

'Patrick says that if the baby comes out half Pakistani, then he will kill me. But he definitely won't let me have an abortion. He says he will never forgive me if I do that. I denied having sex with Kamran, saying it was just petting, but he doesn't believe me. He's right not to believe me! How can I go through months and months of this? What is going to happen at the birth?' Samantha composed herself and spoke slowly, choosing every word carefully. 'Can you help me through this, Dr Leonard? I watch you on TV at breakfast time and you always seem to have answers. I need help and answers. Will you be able to help me?'

'I can't change the course of nature. I'm sure that Patrick doesn't plan to kill you, though – it's just his emotions talking. And, of course, I'll do my best to help get you through this.'

Samantha agreed that Patrick was just showing all his hurt and frustration. 'Patrick has never harmed me before and I can't see anything happening. I think he'll calm down.'

With time, that old enemy, creeping up on us, I decided to get right down to the nitty-gritty. 'What would you like me to do?'

'I had planned to have the baby in hospital but I think it would be better at home with my family around me. If there is an issue over identity I would rather be at home rather than in a public place like a hospital. I just need your support.'

I'm actually quite keen on home births in the right circumstances and this seemed to be one of them. 'Abbey's birth was quite straightforward so you're a good candidate for a home birth. I will arrange all the paper-work, liaise with the midwives and take it from there. You need to have antenatal appointments, as before. But if things don't go according to plan and there are any complications, I would have to advise going into hospital.'

Samantha came to see me over the next few months with updates on her bizarre situation, and she also told me all about her antenatal classes. With the planned home birth a month away, she came in for a check-up and said she had something to ask me.

'Go on,' I encouraged her. 'We've come this far, so I'm sure we can keep moving forward.'

'Will you come along to the birth?'

'There's a really good team of home-birth midwives around here,' I said. 'I know them very well. You'll be in safe hands.'

'But I'd really like you to be there. If you're around it will help to control Patrick's temper.'

'Is he still being threatening?'

'He's still saying he's going to kill me if the baby is "half Paki" as he puts it, but I don't think he really means it . . . I'd still really like you to be there, though.'

I handled lots of deliveries during my five years specialising in obstetrics and gynaecology, and used to do plenty of home births, but times had changed. And, although I was still pretty sure I could deliver a baby if everything went to plan, I was definitely out of practice. It was a job for a skilled midwife who brought babies into the world day in, day out. And to be there as a security consultant wasn't exactly an attractive proposition. I wondered whether I should call social services, but that seemed a bit heavy handed, bearing in mind there had been no abuse so far. And even Samantha didn't believe the threats were genuine. I'd put my heart and soul into her case, though, and Samantha's house was only a few hundred yards from the surgery. I was still concerned about the issue over the father and the patient was pleading with me. 'If I'm free I'll come to the birth, if you really want me to,' I agreed. Apart from anything else I thought it would be a good refresher course for me. 'But I won't be able to come if I'm in the middle of surgery,' I added, reminding myself that I could also be entertaining at home or patching up the chins of neighbouring children.

The bulk of Samantha's antenatal care was carried out, as usual, by the local midwives, but I did see her a couple of times late in her pregnancy. Each time, it struck me that her emotions were flat: she never smiled, had no sense of enjoyment, and was not looking forward to the birth.

I thought she could be depressed and suggested that she talk to one of the specialist teams who deal with mental illness during pregnancy. Tackling her mood before the birth would not only help now, but could also help prevent post-natal depression. And she was a prime candidate for that, especially if the father of her new child proved not to be her husband. But she refused to talk to anyone.

'Counsellors can't tell me the father of my baby, can they? And that's the problem. No, I've just got to see this through, and face the consequences if it turns out badly.'

'How are things with Patrick?'

'Strained. He doesn't talk to me much. I think he's as stressed as I am.'

I sensed she regretted not having a termination. But it was too late for that now. I feared what would happen after the baby was born.

Grace, one of the lovely community midwives, called me on my mobile early on a Friday evening, as I was tidying up and preparing for the weekend.

'Samantha's waters broke this morning. Labour is coming on hard and fast now. It won't be long, I'm sure.'

My last patient disappeared into the evening rush hour, hopefully happy with my advice about the unsightly boils on his bum. It was actually good timing for me to attend the birth – I had nothing planned that evening. I walked the short distance to Samantha's house, enjoying the refreshing spring air and not even objecting to a sudden burst of freezing rain.

I rang the bell and heard Patrick bellowing, 'It's open, come on up.'

I felt the tension as soon as I opened the heavy, rustic, wooden door. Patrick had obviously carried out a lot of the work on this, one of the older properties in the area. The door opened to reveal another glass door inside the porch and then I walked into the lounge where Samantha's daughter, Abbey, was sitting playing a computer game.

'Hello,' she grinned. 'It's all happening upstairs.' Yes, I thought, I can hear the unmistakable noises of a woman in labour. I had arrived just in time, with my head full of thoughts about the baby's appearance. Was Patrick the father? Did the baby belong to Kamran? How would Patrick react if the baby wasn't his?

As I stepped into the bedroom, I saw that Samantha was clearly in the third, pushing stage of labour. She was lying on the bed, her head propped up on several pillows, all with different patterned covers, and the mattress and bottom sheet were protected with a large piece of plastic. Grace had everything neatly arranged. I could see the instruments she needed and the gauze swabs all laid out at the foot of the bed.

After every contraction, Samantha's face contorted with a mix of pain and effort, and she screamed as she pushed the baby down through her pelvis. Patrick stood beside the bed, holding her hand. He was a large man, with huge arm muscles, and I hoped fervently that he didn't mean what he had said about killing his wife. Neither Grace nor I would have stood a chance against him. But I was relieved to see he had dark brown hair. It would have been potentially far more difficult if he'd been blond or ginger. As it was, even if the baby had dark hair, there was a chance that it could be Patrick's baby.

With the next push Grace and I could see the top of the baby's head appear at the entrance of Samantha's vagina. My heart sank as I saw the baby's black hair. I feared the worst. This couldn't be Patrick's child, could it? But, with the next contraction, the face appeared, and I saw a ruddy pink Caucasian colour. I breathed a sigh of relief. The baby was Patrick's, after all. Next came the shoulders and then, with a final gentle push, a beautiful baby boy greeted the world. It was only when I looked at his scrotum that I realised who the father really was. I was hoping to see a dark red scrotum, but this little chap's was far darker than is normal for a Caucasian boy. Both Grace and I could see from this that the baby had a strong Asian connection. The question was, as I held my breath, had Patrick noticed this, too?

The room fell silent; nine months of tension filled the room. Patrick stared at the new arrival. Grace tidied up and mopped Samantha's brow. And I sweated and kept quiet.

'My darling, what a lovely baby,' Patrick yelled, hugging his wife. 'This is my gorgeous new son. Welcome to our family!' Patrick clearly believed that the baby was his own flesh and blood. 'Samantha, I am so sorry. I am so sorry. I should have known the baby was mine all along.' He then whispered in his wife's ear and I could just detect a string of apologies; he was prepared to accept that her other relationship had just been 'friendly'.

With mother and baby united, and Grace and I happy with their health, Samantha began breastfeeding. I winked at the new mum and made my way back to the surgery for more tidying up before the weekend.

I wondered what would happen as the years passed. Surely the boy's Asian parentage would become more obvious. How would Patrick react then?

As the boy grew up, his heritage did become more obvious, confirming my suspicions. He had very dark hair, although his skin was still light. But when he was brought to the surgery, by either Samantha or Patrick, all seemed to be well. Amazingly, they were an extremely happy family. Patrick clearly loved him like his own son; even if he suspected that he wasn't the father, he never said a word. And Samantha seemed happy, and never mentioned her troubled pregnancy again.

I never knew what happened to Kamran, or whether Samantha had any more contact with him. I certainly wasn't going to bring the issue up when I saw her. I did wonder, though, what would happen when the boy was older. From a medical viewpoint, knowing about diseases which run in your family, such as heart conditions, can be very important. And then there is the emotional part of knowing your heritage. But, for now, that house was filled with love again, and I was more than happy to let them all get on with their lives.

Back in the surgery, though, there were more issues over identity . . .

'Hello, Sally, what can I do for you?' I asked as a

familiar face came in. Instead of her usual smile, though, her face was downcast and her eyes were moist with tears, smudging her mascara.

'I've just found out that my mother died while giving birth to me.'

'Oh, I'm so sorry,' I said, completely taken by surprise. No wonder she looked so upset. 'How on earth did you find out?'

'It all came out about a year ago. To begin with, I thought I could cope, but I now know that I can't.' Tears flowed down Sally's cheeks. 'I think I need some help.'

As Sally sat there, tears streaming from her puffy eyes down her cheeks, I tried to get my head around the dramatic change in family circumstances. Sally was only twenty; the woman, known to me as her mother, was really her stepmother. I knew the family fairly well. They had moved into the area to allow the children to go to the local private schools. I could see that she didn't appear to share any of the physical traits of the woman I'd assumed to be her mother but her father was an occasional patient and I could see the resemblance there. She had her father's nose and the same high cheekbones.

Sally was totally distraught and I decided that it would help if she told me the whole story. After that I thought I would be able to work out the best way of helping her. Her experience was quite remarkable; I was glued to her story from start to finish.

'I found out after watching a TV programme,' Sally explained.

'A TV programme?' I said, genuinely keen to find out more. 'How did that happen?'

'Well, it was that programme, *Who Do You Think You Are?* And I watched it because my favourite celebrity was appearing. You know the programme – it's where the celeb finds out about family roots.'

'Yes, I like that programme. It's made me want to know more about my ancestors.'

'And that's just what happened to me. I found out about my family history.' More tears appeared in Sally's eyes as she continued. 'I was sitting watching the programme with my father and I told him that I was fascinated by family history. I asked him all about our family, whether there were any illnesses over the years and that sort of thing. I wanted to know everything.'

I noticed that she was leaving long pauses as she told her story. She was one of those people who weighed up what they were going to say carefully. She was an intelligent young woman, on the short side with black, close-cropped hair and a face that changed expression every few seconds.

'So he told you everything?'

'My dad walked over to the telly and switched it off,' Sally continued. 'He held my hand and looked me straight in the eyes. Mummy, or the person I've always known as Mummy but who isn't really, wasn't in the room. She was upstairs with the others – my brother and sister. Well, I've always thought that they were my brother and sister but they're actually my half-brother and half-sister . . .' There was a pause. I decided to wait for her until she was ready to continue her extraordinary story. 'Daddy said he had wanted to tell me about my background for years, but the opportunity never arose.' Sally's father then told her how his wife had died while giving birth. He and the rest of the family had been traumatised and needed counselling. 'I survived the birth and, to begin with, my mother's parents looked after me. Then, when I was around one year old, Dad met someone else – my future stepmother, the woman I know as Mummy – and they were married.'

'Why didn't he tell you sooner? Eighteen years is a long time to keep a secret like that.'

'Well, he said he had always wanted to tell me but he kept putting it off. As the years went by, he found it more and more difficult to say anything about it. To be fair, Mummy, or my stepmother, treated me like one of her own so I have no complaints there. I just thought she was my biological mother.'

'I'm surprised you didn't find out from someone else.'

Sally cried a little and then composed herself. 'Yes, but everyone was sworn to secrecy. Both sets of grandparents said nothing and, of course, when my stepmother had two more children I assumed that they were my brother and sister. Well, they were my dad's children but you know what I mean.'

I knew what she meant. Sally was kept in the dark because the entire family had agreed to say nothing for the sake of unity. What if Sally had rejected her new mother? Although it all made sense, I felt that Sally should have been told the truth several years ago.

'I was the only child of my biological mother. You can see that my stepmother had a completely different family tree. What a nightmare. And it's been awful for my genuine maternal grandparents. Daddy kept in touch with them, but in order to keep the secret I never saw them. I have met them now, but of course they were like strangers at first.'

Sally burst into tears once more. I let her get it all out of her system for a few moments before suggesting a plan of action. I asked what she knew about her real mother.

'It was so hard for me. Once the secret was out, my father produced a hoard of pictures from the loft. He is still a dentist, as you know, and my real mum worked as an administrator at the council. I was amazed that he had been married before and never told me. It was as if my mum had never existed.' Sally was eager to fill me in on the rest of her story. 'I discovered where she was buried but how do you mourn someone you never knew? I discovered all I could about her and did all sorts of family tree checks, just like the programme on telly. The positive part about all this is that everyone knows the truth and we can all talk about it.'

I wondered how Sally's stepmother had adapted and asked how that relationship was working. 'She's kept the secret for a long time, too, and brought you up as her own child – has it been hard for her?'

'Mummy – though it seems odd calling her that now – has been simply amazing,' Sally reflected. 'The strain was getting to her as well. She always wanted to tell me the truth but my dad held off and held off. Deep down, she felt it was important for the family to discuss what had happened and move on.'

'Right,' I agreed. 'Everyone is moving on.'

'Everyone except me,' she started sobbing again. 'I can't move on. Apart from thinking about my real mother all of the time, I have an irrational fear of having children. I'm terrified. I'm terrified I'll die just like my own mother. What if I plan to settle down? I won't be able to have kids. I'm too scared. I mean, I'm seeing someone at the moment. What if we build a relationship and I can't have children?'

The pain was etched on Sally's face. It wasn't surprising really that she had found it so difficult. She was going through a mix of shock and bereavement. There are several stages of bereavement and, despite the time delay, she would experience them all. Firstly, she would have to accept that her loss was real; she would have to experience the pain of grief; she needed to adjust to the dramatic change in her life; and then hopefully she would be able to 'move on'. That would mean putting less emotional energy into grieving and dwelling on the past, and more effort into the present. A new sport or hobby can often prove helpful.

I know from personal experience that grief can turn your life upside down. Your personality, beliefs and emotions are all affected. Some people, including Sally, find it difficult to adjust to the immense changes in everyday life. There is no standard time limit; everyone copes in his or her own way. Some mourners become withdrawn, others turn completely numb and a few experience the serious issues of depression.

'Have you thought about bereavement counselling?' I suggested. 'It might just help you to adjust to all the changes in your life. You'll have to accept the loss, and everything associated with it, before you can move forward. In the end, hopefully you will come to accept what has happened.'

'Would it really help me?' Sally asked as more tears appeared on her cheeks. 'I am doing some odd things. I've lost my purse twice today and I've just remembered that I have a lunch appointment.'

'That can happen during emotional shock and bereavement,' I assured Sally. 'It can make people forgetful and that seems to have happened to you.'

Sally smiled and I could tell that an enormous weight was about to be taken off her shoulders. 'I'll give it a try. I suppose bereavement counselling can't do any harm.'

Several months later, Sally reappeared in my surgery to give me an update; what a transformation. The lines that once helped tears to flow down her cheeks now formed a weak – although distinct – smile.

'How are you?' I enquired. 'Are you feeling any better?'

'I had problems with the counselling to start with. I saw an older woman and she did her best. For a while the thought of never knowing my mum really got to me. I was so angry because no one had ever told me about her. It took a while to ease that anger out of me.'

'Are you still angry?' I asked, hoping that all the resentment had gone.

'Just a little. The counsellor was used to dealing with people who had had some sort of relationship with their loved one. In my case, I never even knew that my mother existed so I was a rather unique case.'

'How do you feel about everything now?'

Sally explained how she had more or less come to terms with her loss. 'That anger did prove to be a stumbling block, but time is also a great healer. That is definitely true. The counsellor explored all the areas which were preventing me from moving on and addressed them one by one.'

I was impressed with the bereavement counsellor's work. Sally had, at last, accepted her situation and was ready to get on with her life. 'You certainly do look a totally different person,' I observed. 'When you came in here last time you were in a real state. I've dealt with quite a few unique situations in my time, and yours is one of them, for sure.'

'Oh, just one thing,' Sally added. 'After talking everything through so much and looking at all the issues, I'm not so scared now. I think I'm ready.'

I wasn't sure what she meant. 'Ready? What are you ready for?'

'I'm ready to have kids, if my partner agrees. The counselling has removed that fear – and for that, I will be grateful for the rest of my life.'

We both stood up and I gave Sally a gentle doctor-to-patient hug.

My daily routine involves more than handing out pills and sending swabs off for tests. I see my job as helping my family of patients under any circumstances.

I wouldn't have it any other way.

CHAPTER TEN

HEATHER AND CASSANDRA

'I think I saw a patient of yours in town over the weekend,' Naz told me as we sat down together with our cups of tea. 'I was enjoying a special night out for my parents' wedding anniversary, and we were at a really good restaurant – far more expensive than the ones we usually go to. She was looking amazingly glam. I don't live on the patch like you do, so I find it a bit weird when I see patients when I'm off duty, especially at a place like that. And they look so different – you know how they normally look when they come in here.'

'I don't suppose you remember her name?'

'No, I'm nearly as bad as you with names. I can usually remember what's wrong with a patient, but often can't remember what they are called.'

'I wonder who that could have been,' I pondered as we studied the agenda for the early evening doctors' meeting.

'My newspaper didn't arrive this morning,' Dr David butted in brusquely. 'You know it has a feature on sixty-five years of the NHS and I haven't been able to read it. Did you know that the NHS has been going for sixty-five years?'

'You should get it online,' Naz pointed out. 'Then it would be sure to arrive and you wouldn't fill up the recycling bag getting rid of it. The recycling is mostly made up of your newspapers.'

'I spend all day here glued to a computer screen,' Dr David exploded. 'There is no way I want to read my morning paper on it as well. Some things are, well, sacred, I'll have you know.'

'And you wouldn't end up with newspaper print all over your fingers,' Naz continued.

'Online? No way. All I want is my newspaper!'

'I'm sure Lizzy can check with the newsagent to find out what happened,' I added, trying to keep the peace.

'I heard that,' Lizzy smiled as she appeared with more tea on a tray. 'Haud yer wheesht. The paper didn't come this morning. Maybe they were still writing that NHS story after sixty-five years. I bet you worked for the NHS sixty-five years ago, David.'

'Ha, ha,' Dr David laughed out loud. 'Haud yer what? Are you speaking in a foreign language?'

Lizzy apologised for breaking into her native Scottish tongue. 'It means that you must be quiet when I'm talking. You know that I start using Scottish phrases when I'm cross!'

Our proud Scottish receptionist flicked back her long black hair and gave us a flash of those dazzling blue eyes. 'And, talking of computers, I need to check you lot are using the correct codes for recording smoking and blood pressure. Having those codes is the only way I can run reports, and we are still way down on our targets.'

David groaned. 'It's not enough to make patients better, or even keep them well these days, is it? We've got to record every last fact about them so some politician can claim the government has managed to cut smoking rates. As if the government has done anything about smoking. It's us who have to do the work . . .'

We all agreed that QOF, the abbreviation for Quality and Outcomes Framework, was making our lives as GPs a bit of a misery. It was designed to make sure all GPs provided high-quality care to their patients by giving them a financial incentive for making sure we asked the right questions and carried out important tests. There was no doubt that, for some people with long-term conditions such as diabetes or asthma, care had definitely improved.

'I know, I know but just remember that recording that data helps to pay for my salary, and for that chocolate biscuit you're about to eat,' Lizzy added, seeing his hand stray towards the heavily laden plate.

'Sorry, I'm just a bit weary of computers,' David apologised. 'My whole working life these days seems to revolve around QOF. I hardly seem to look at my patients any more. And when I do it's to ask ridiculous questions. I had to ask a ninety-three-year-old today how many hours a week she spent riding a bicycle, for God's sake. I do believe she thought I'd lost the plot.'

To begin with, QOF only accounted for a small proportion of the income coming into the practice but now, as Lizzy had reminded us, it was vital for paying the salaries of several of our members of staff. With extra tests and questions to ask, the money was even more difficult to obtain. We genuinely could not afford to ignore the tick boxes.

Our regular monthly early evening brainstorming sessions in Dr David's consulting room were worthwhile exercises; any issues could be raised and problems were usually solved, including dealing with Dr David's ever-growing list of moans about how general practice was changing for the worse.

'Tell me more about the patient you saw,' I quizzed Naz as we locked the surgery front door. 'You mentioned the glam one. I'm wondering who she is.'

'Tall and very good looking. Wonderful posture. In the last year I've seen her come in quite often to see you. Apart from that I don't know anything about her – except that she was with a gent who appeared to be an Arab businessman. We did wonder what the relationship was between them – if you know what I mean . . .'

'Eh?'

'Well, my dad thought she might be a high-class hooker. He said she had "that look" about her, whatever he meant by that.'

I agreed that I probably wouldn't recognise a high-class prostitute either, and we laughed as we said our goodbyes for the evening and drove off in our cars.

The next morning, I wondered again who Naz was on about. Was one of my regular patients really working as a prostitute? If so, I fervently hoped they were practising safe sex. Usually, I had some evidence to work with or a few ideas to help with difficult situations. All I had to go on was a vague notion from Naz that another unusual set of circumstances was heading in my direction.

I dealt with constipation, a mysterious rash, a flourishing wart and a bout of flu before Heather arrived in the surgery.

'Good morning,' I greeted my patient of at least seven years. 'I haven't seen you for a while. Any problems?'

'Just a check on my sexual health. You can't be too careful these days, if you know what I mean. I just like the occasional check-up.'

I recalled several similar requests from other patients. 'Well, I can carry out the tests, but there are specialised clinics who can give you much quicker results. It's up to you, really. I have to send off your samples and wait for the results.'

'I know they do a top job,' she replied, 'but with my work and everything, I would be happier just coming to see you.'

I accepted that explanation. After all, Heather worked in the corporate hospitality business, and, like many others, I understood that she did not really want to be spotted in a genito-urinary clinic. Even in today's open society, many felt there was a stigma attached to going there, that you were being labelled as promiscuous – which was nonsense, of course. I knew that she was a single mother; her husband had run off with another woman when their daughter, now nine, was three years old. Looking at Heather's records, I could see that she had just celebrated her thirty-fifth birthday. She still had finely sculpted features and more than a touch of class about her. Heather had obviously come from a privileged background. She used the clipped vowels and diction of the English upper classes and said 'crikey-o' every second or third sentence. She was the only patient I knew who said 'crikey-o'!

I carried out the necessary tests and watched as Heather strutted across the consulting room. She must have been taught deportment, because she glided across the room with her back straight and her head held high, showing her full height of almost six feet, even in flat ballet pumps. I noticed that her tight, skinny trousers showed off a fabulous figure. I admired her natural, long, flowing, blonde hair.

On previous visits, with track suits and sporting gear, she'd looked athletic. Now, I could tell as she headed off to work, that a highly attractive, fairly young lady – leaving behind a trail of expensive-smelling scent – had just left my surgery.

Her tests were clear but, a month later, Heather was back. 'I just need some more checks. Crikey-o, you can't be too careful, can you? You never know what you can pick up.'

I did wonder why Heather needed so many sexual health checks. However, she explained that she was just being ultra-careful and, of course, I accepted what she was saying. She mentioned one or two slight issues down below so I asked her to get up on the couch and I took some swabs.

'Is everything all right?' I asked during that second visit. 'You seem to be a little downcast, if you don't mind me saying.'

'No, I don't mind,' she answered, staring at the floor. 'I am struggling at the moment because my ex-husband is playing up again.'

'Playing up? I remember that he left you for someone else. You told me that a few years ago. In what way is he playing up?'

Heather's mood changed as she divulged a copious amount of ill-feeling towards her ex-partner. Her face twisted with hatred as she explained their situation. 'He's not giving me any money,' she hissed. 'He's still working – self-employed as a music teacher travelling around the country – but he's got around the child maintenance rule and is giving me hardly anything. It's barely enough to buy food for myself and Charlotte.'

'That sort of behaviour makes me so cross,' I admitted. 'It's so unfair on women.'

While Heather held her head in her hands, I also cursed her former partner for getting around the child maintenance system. He should have been paying fifteen per cent of his net income, but had found ways of declaring tiny earnings.

'Is there nothing you can do to get some money out of him?'

Heather shook her head. 'His parents have got some money, but I really don't want to involve them and, anyway, they are likely to take his side, aren't they? I've received some forms to fill in but they're horrible-looking things. I've got to rush off now. I'll give you an update when I come back again.'

Come back again, I thought? I was intrigued. It was no trouble to take some samples and swabs and send them off to the lab, but I did wonder what was going on. She hadn't mentioned a new boyfriend. Also, she preferred to come in for the results as soon as I had them. She wanted to see me rather than discuss results over the phone. I did begin to wonder whether she could be the high-class prostitute that Naz had mentioned.

'Is everything all clear?' Heather asked as she made yet another appearance a few days later. 'You know that soreness and discharge I had? Was that anything to worry about?'

'It's thrush,' I responded in matter-of-fact style. 'It's an infection caused by a yeast fungus. It's very common. It tends to occur when there is a change in your natural protective secretions inside your vagina, and it doesn't take much for your system to get out of balance.'

Heather looked relieved. 'Yes, I've had that type of thing before. I didn't get it from having sex, then?'

'Well, it can be sexually transmitted, but actually that's quite rare. It may be linked to an increase in sexual activity, though. What normally happens is that the vagina can be irritated during sex, or the acidity levels can change, allowing thrush to grow more than usual. The itchy discharge you have can be treated easily with anti-fungal pessaries. I'm sure that will sort things out.'

'I didn't get it from sex, then,' Heather asked me again.

'It's unlikely. So many things can change conditions inside your vagina. You have more chance of developing thrush if you wear tight clothing that prevents ventilation. Some people use a vaginal deodorant or a perfumed bubble bath, and these can cause irritation. It's nothing serious.'

Off she went again, seemingly satisfied with my

explanation. I carried on with my other appointments, ranging from a follow-up on that annoying wart to a vast array of aches and pains. During quiet moments, my mind wandered back to Heather, the errant ex-husband and her continual check-ups.

The weekend drew nearer and a girls' night out I had planned began to appear on the horizon. I'd been in contact with some old friends from my Cambridge days and we were going to have a trip down memory lane. The taxi was expected at seven o'clock sharp on Saturday evening. I enjoyed the excuse to dress up. I had arranged to meet Sophie and Mary at a wine bar in Pimlico; as they were arriving from different locations, it made sense to meet somewhere in the centre of town.

They had booked into a local hotel and I wasn't driving, so a marvellous evening lay in store. I treated myself to a glass of wine while I waited for the taxi.

I looked in the mirror and saw, hopefully, something approaching a pillar of society; a healer of all ailments; a wart expert; a medical detective; a total workaholic; and a GP dressed in slightly better garb than my usual surgery clothes. I told the rest of the family where I was going, said to call me if needed, and breezed off in the taxi for the short ride to Pimlico.

This doctor in patent, black, high heels, wearing a well-fitting, dark purple dress, with hair and make-up sorted out, couldn't wait to see her old pals.

I felt good as I strode into the wine bar; I was a few

minutes early and slipped into a comfy armchair in the corner. A large rubbery plant kept me partly hidden from Dr Rosemary Leonard fans. I needed a night off from treating patients and giving out advice.

The sight that met my eyes when I sat down was totally beyond belief, though. I could see on a stool at the bar a face that I knew very well indeed. But everything about Heather caught me by surprise. She was wearing what appeared to be expensive designer gear from head to toe. Of course, I had seen her in business clothes and also in sporty attire, but this was a complete transformation.

The woman at the bar, drinking champagne from an elegant flute, was an entirely different proposition. She wore an expensive-looking blue dress, around knee length, just showing a hint of her cleavage. She wore tasteful bracelets and earrings – nothing ostentatious – and these blended in perfectly with her blue outfit. She wore black, open-toed sandals, showing off her perfect feet and freshly painted, subtle pink toenails. She looked beautiful, sexy and sophisticated all at once.

Heather sat only about ten feet away, trying to look in the opposite direction. Although I was dressed to the hilt, I felt that, on this occasion, Heather had the edge. But what was she doing here? Who was she meeting?

'Hello, I'm Darren,' a voice said behind me. 'Very pleased to meet you.'

'Hi, I'm Cassandra,' I could hear Heather reply.

Cassandra? Eh? What was going on? What was Heather doing here dressed up to the nines? Who was she with? Why had she changed her name? Was she earning money in a rather dubious way? Then I remembered my conversation with Naz. Was Heather really the mysterious patient from the restaurant who her father had labelled a high-class prostitute? Looking at her in the bar she certainly looked high class but, maybe naively, I found it difficult to believe that she was 'on the game'.

I sat tight, hoping she hadn't noticed me but, unfortunately, the earlier glass of wine ensured that a visit to the loo was necessary. It was still a few minutes before I was expecting my two friends, and they had a reputation for always being late in our student days. The toilets were perilously close to the bar. I tried hard to avoid Heather and I almost made it, head down, in the direction of the ladies, but our eyes met. It was the briefest of glances.

When I returned from the toilet, Cassandra and her 'date' were gone. Replacing the odd couple at the bar I could see Sophie and Mary, both thirty years older but instantly recognisable. We hugged and we hugged until the hugging session threatened to become embarrassing.

'I see you're doing well on the telly, then,' Sophie said in her strong Welsh accent. 'You're in the newspapers, too. I'm still tending to my flock in the valleys, but no one has asked me to go on the telly.'

Mary gave her friend a disapproving look. 'She's only

jealous,' she said in her posh accent. 'Her patients are farmers with a few sheep. It was so quiet last week that one of the sheep made an appointment.'

'Hey you, lay off,' Sophie bit back. 'Just because you deal with all the posh people of Oxford, you think you've made it. You're not in the real world among that lot. The real, hard-working GPs are down in my neck of the woods.'

'Girls, girls,' I interrupted. 'I see nothing has changed. I'm sure we are all working flat-out. Shall we have a drink and do some catching up?'

As I chatted to Sophie and Mary, memories of our student days came flooding back. Most of our memories revolved around our nights out in Cambridge in the distant seventies when we were studying and partying at the same time. Fortunately we were able to knuckle down during the serious days and we successfully pushed for the highest grades possible.

'What a day that was at Cherry Hinton Hall,' Mary remembered. 'Cambridge Folk Festival, eh? What a bash that was. I went along just to see Tom Rush playing "No Regrets". He was fantastic, wasn't he, Rosemary?'

'Oh yes, he was just amazing,' I fibbed, flicking back through the years in my mind. 'It wasn't in a hall, though. I seem to remember a lot of people in a field? And that you had to drag me there?' Folk festivals weren't really my scene then, or now. I much prefer going to the Proms.

The banter with my friends continued, as we enjoyed a meal at the wine bar. I forgot all about my mysterious patient with her changing name but a week later, I noticed a familiar name on my appointments list for the day. Heather had arranged another check-up.

Her private life was her own and I had no intention of making any observations or stirring things up.

'I know you saw me in the wine bar,' Heather said with a hint of a smile as soon as she appeared for her appointment. 'You must have wondered what I was doing there – and I think you heard that I used a different name. I'm not proud of myself – quite the opposite, in fact. I feel really embarrassed, especially when I recognise someone. However, at the moment, I have no choice.'

If she wanted to tell me, then I was prepared to listen. 'I'm just here to treat you as your GP. I can't tell you how to run your personal life, but please share your problems with me.'

'You've probably guessed, so I may as well be honest with you,' she continued. 'I work as an escort,' Heather confided. 'I'm with a good agency and the work pays really good money. In theory, I'm just supposed to have dinner with the men, or be their companion for the evening, but I get paid a lot more if I have sex with them.'

Heather was in full flow, and I allowed her to continue without interruption.

'As you can guess, most of them want sex. My job

salary just doesn't cover the bills. I've tried to think of alternatives, but this is the only way I can pay the mortgage and the bills, not to mention the school fees. Charlotte is bright and I want the best for her. And my family would be horrified if she went to a state school . . .' They'd be horrified if they knew what you were doing, I thought to myself. Was her daughter's private education really worth the sale of her body? She clearly thought so. 'I hate doing it. You saw that tiny bloke, Darren, with the odd moustache. Well, that's a typical date for me. Wasn't he horrible?'

'I didn't really catch sight of him,' I lied. 'Anyway, I can see now why you come here for all those tests!'

'I always take along a pack of condoms. We're supposed to refuse sex if they won't wear one, but none of the clients want to wear them, really. The tiny bloke with the moustache brought his own condom, but he had such a tiny cock that I hardly noticed a thing.'

'I can picture the scene,' I chortled, wondering whether the small man had more to offer than my 'disappearing penis' patient.

'Do you think I am at risk of catching something serious?' Heather asked, with a worried expression.

'In a word, yes. You just don't know where these people have been. I would suggest always using your own condom, so you can be sure they are a decent strength. Goodness knows where your clients' condoms come from. They could easily be cheap ones that tear or burst.

I wouldn't trust anything like that. Bring your own and insist that they wear it.'

'I have to be firmer,' Heather said, sternly, and I grinned. 'Sorry,' she laughed. 'That was a bad, or maybe a good, choice of word.'

'Possibly appropriate,' I smiled.

'But,' Heather continued, as her face suddenly became more serious, 'a couple of weeks ago one of the clients became quite aggressive and insisted on sex without a condom. He was an older businessman, a bit smelly and quite aggressive. I was sore the next day because he was such a turn-off that I didn't get excited in the slightest.'

'Aren't your clients screened in any way?' I asked, concerned at the latest development.

'The agency does that. They find out as much as possible. But you can never tell what someone is going to be like on a one-to-one basis. I always carry a pepper spray just in case. I haven't had to use it, but I have it with me at all times. My phone is always switched on, too, so I can call for help quickly. The escort business is legal, but I'm not sure if I should be carrying weapons.'

'Sounds like a hazardous occupation,' I said.

'I was safe enough the other night. The strange little bloke paid me £750 in cash. I always get the money up front to avoid any problems later. That was an easy job, especially as he wore a condom and it was all over in around five minutes. The money went straight into the bank the following day.'

Heather and Cassandra

I didn't approve of the lifestyle but I had to admire Heather's determination to keep her daughter at a private school despite her ex-husband's hopeless payment record. I was fascinated to hear about Heather's night job, but kept stressing the health risks.

'How often are you doing this?'

'It's usually about twice a week, sometimes three times, but no more than that.'

I did some quick mental sums in my head. She was earning at least £1,500 a week, sometimes more. But for that she was having sex with umpteen different men, and sometimes it was unprotected.

She had her serious face on again. 'I'm rather concerned about my client this coming Friday night. I agreed to see him, despite a few problems last time.'

'What sort of problems?'

'I met him in that wine bar a few weeks ago, he gave me £1,000 in cash, and we went off to a local hotel. Part of the deal was that he didn't have to wear a condom. I wasn't happy about it, but an extra £250 is always useful. And I seem to be OK, health wise, because of the time that's passed.'

I knew I'd taken a full set of swabs in the past fortnight, so I wasn't concerned about a vaginal infection, but now I'd heard her story I realised there were other tests that needed to be done.

'Heather, while you are doing this job you must have regular blood tests as well for syphilis, hepatitis B and HIV.'

'Hepatitis B? HIV? I thought only gays got those?'
She sounded horrified.

'It's true that the majority of cases are in men who
have sex with men, but lots of cases occur in women, too.
You don't know who those men have had sex with before
you. They could be carrying anything.' She looked really
scared as I wrote out the blood form. 'You can go and get
this done at the local hospital,' I instructed her. 'I don't
need to put the reason why. We do loads of them, so
there's no need to be embarrassed. But we don't give the
results out over the phone. Make an appointment to see
me in a week. The results should be back by then. I know
you say you need the money but, really, you shouldn't be
putting your health at risk with any bloke, no matter how
much he's paying. Insist they wear a condom,' I stressed.
'Please. Otherwise you could be risking an illness that
will stay with you for the rest of your life.'

'It's not so much the condom that's worrying me. He
wants me to go to his house. What should I do? Crikey-o,
I don't know.'

That sounded a very dodgy idea to me, and I said so.
I knew little about the escort business but I reckoned
hotels had to be safer than private homes.

'He said he wanted to try other things. He's asked me
to wear black, lace-up boots . . .'

Oh help, I thought, surely she's not going to ask my
advice about the safety of S & M sex. That was a topic
that medical school didn't cover.

'No,' I told her firmly, aware I was sounding rather prim. 'As you're asking me, I have to say no, no, no all day long.'

'I'll get another £1,000 in cash,' she reminded me, almost pleading for my approval.

'I'm just your GP, not a counsellor or adviser but, as you asked me, I have to say it all sounds risky.'

'You're right,' Heather nodded. 'I'll put him off and meet the guy you saw in the wine bar. He only pays £750, but it will be in a hotel and I hardly have to work for it. He won't pay the £1,000, but I feel safe with him, even if it is a horrible experience.'

'Good idea,' I agreed. 'If you take any chances, you will need your regular check-ups. Bye, Cassandra . . . sorry, I mean, Heather.'

'I'm Heather today,' she grinned. 'I'll be Cassandra on Friday night. In fact, I'll be Cassandra on most weekends while Charlotte is at that posh expensive school.'

'Safety first,' I reminded her, 'and I'll see you next week.'

Thankfully the blood tests were negative and Heather and I agreed that I would see her for checks once a month for swabs, and once every three months for blood tests. She was happy to see me more often if any symptoms appeared. Every time I saw her it was clear that she loathed what she was doing, but it was the best way she could find of paying her bills and maintaining the lifestyle she and her daughter were accustomed to.

I did worry about her long-term mental health and how her daughter would feel if she ever found out how her education had been paid for. But Heather always took a pragmatic line. 'Loads of people are out there kissing and shagging anyway. Look at the number of people who do Internet dating. I just make sure I get paid for it. And the moment I've got the bills covered, I'm going to give it up.'

I saw her on and off for the next two years. She appeared to have taken my advice about condoms, because the swabs and blood tests mercifully remained clear. Then, one day, she walked in with a large bunch of lilies.

'These are for you,' she said, handing them over. 'I wanted to say thank you for looking after me.' I wondered what was coming next. 'You see, I won't need to come to see you so often any more. I paid the mortgage off last week and I've enough money in the bank to cover the school fees. So I can now have my Friday and Saturday nights to myself.'

'You're giving it up?'

'Absolutely. I always said I would. I've sold my body for long enough. But I've no regrets. I'll even be able to buy a decent house in the country once Charlotte has left school. And, thanks to you, I've come to no physical harm.'

'And mentally?' I had to ask. 'What about relationships? Do you think you'll ever have a partner again?'

'I doubt it. I never say never but, crikey-o, I've lost all respect for men. First there was my ex and, since then, I've come across all sorts of oddballs who just want to pay for sex. And, quite frankly, I've seen enough willies to last me a lifetime. I really don't want to see, let alone feel, another one in a long, long time.' I could understand where she was coming from. The life she had chosen had taken its toll. 'For me, sex has just become a means to a financial end. I can't ever imagine connecting it with feelings. And I've become an ace at faking an orgasm.'

My mind wandered back to *When Harry Met Sally.* 'Better than the movie?'

'Oh yes. Much quicker, too. Makes the man feel he's some sort of expert, and I get to go home a bit quicker. They never seem to realise . . .'

'Well, give it time. You are still young,' I reminded her. 'Maybe in a couple of years you'll think differently. And, if you ever want to see a counsellor, or talk to someone about it, you know where to come.'

'The only person I've ever spoken to about this is you, Rosemary. You've been so supportive. I can't thank you enough, especially since you haven't been judgemental. But if I need any more help, I will be back.'

As she left, I thought of my sons. As a single mother I, too, had worked all hours to earn enough to provide for them, but for me the price had just been losing sleep, not self-respect.

As Heather hurried out of the surgery and into her

car, Naz peered round my door. 'Is she all right? I saw her in town again during one of my famous nights out, but didn't want to say anything. I just reckoned that you were in for a few surprises there and it was none of my business.'

'I have had a few surprises,' I grinned. 'Thanks for keeping everything to yourself. She's done amazing things to keep her daughter in school.'

'Best not to tell me,' Naz said. 'Some mothers will go to the ends of the earth to look after their children. It baffles me why so many fathers try so hard to get out of paying their share. It's always the children who suffer in the end.'

'Hopefully her daughter will be OK, as long as she never finds out how her fees were paid. When you go out to reception, would you mind telling Lizzy that I'm ready for my next patient?'

As I remembered again all the details of Heather's bizarre case, I thought to myself: good luck, Cassandra. And crikey-o!

CHAPTER ELEVEN

THE TURKEY BASTER

I was looking forward to a few normal, routine days when Ellen appeared in the surgery.

I'd known Ellen for a year or so. She worked in the media – I was never sure exactly what that entailed – and she looked the type. In the summer she wore tight jeans or loose linen trousers, designer trainers and T-shirts. In the winter she was smothered in colourful, baggy jumpers, which looked capable of accommodating three or more Ellens.

Ellen turned up for her appointment as early autumn leaves swirled around outside, and everything looked baggy. Her shirt and trousers flopped around her as she sat in the chair.

'I'm getting a bit bloated,' she groaned, pointing to her stomach. 'It's intermittent. Sometimes I get diarrhoea and at other times I'm constipated. I don't really know what's going on. My previous doctor said I had Irritable Bowel Syndrome. Do you think it's getting worse?'

I agreed to check that there was nothing more serious going on. She had no blood in her motions; she hadn't lost any weight; and seemed to be well enough otherwise. She appeared rather stressed, though, and I knew that would only make her condition flare up. With IBS the muscles in the bowel that control the passage of faeces do not work in the normal co-ordinated way. Instead some sections of the large bowel muscle go into spasm, causing pain, while others relax, leading to bloating.

I carried out some routine blood tests to check that she wasn't anaemic or had any problems with her kidneys or liver. I checked her ESR level, or Erythrocyte Sedimentation Rate, via a blood test. It measures abnormal protein levels which can indicate inflammation in the body. ESR can be raised in many inflammatory conditions such as abscesses, arthritis and cancers. Levels of ESR are usually higher in females and, as people get older, the levels tend to increase. It's a very general test, but if levels are raised it can be an indication that some more specific investigations need to be carried out.

I also asked Ellen to produce a stool sample to test for infection, blood, and other markers, which could be an indication that her bowel lining was inflamed. This would be a sign that the problem was not IBS – as that doesn't cause inflammation. I also asked her to keep a detailed food diary to see if I could track down the reason for the bloating. Although the exact cause of IBS isn't known, it is sometimes linked to eating certain types of food, such as onions, especially in large amounts.

'I believe I've worked out what was causing the bloating,' Ellen said, smugly, when she reappeared a couple of weeks later. 'I eat large amounts of onions, leeks and broccoli.'

'Those are known culprits,' I confirmed.

'I kept my detailed diary, noticed that those vegetables played an enormous part in my diet and so I cut them down. Now the bloating has more or less gone. I still have some abdominal pain and cramping, a bit too much wind for my partner's liking and occasional urgent needs to go to the toilet.'

'Do you get anxious or depressed?' I asked.

'No, I don't seem to have any of that. I just feel a lot of stress. I write articles for magazines for a living and am always rushing to meet deadlines, which is stressful – as you will know only too well!'

'I can back that up,' I said with a knowing grin. I often end up writing my column at the last minute. 'I was curious about whether you felt anxious or depressed, though, because three out of four people with IBS will have at least one bout of depression. More than half will have generalised anxiety disorder. I just had to rule those out. There is no cure for IBS,' I explained. 'However, changes to your lifestyle can relieve a lot of the symptoms.'

Doctor's Notes

I told Ellen to have regular meals, taking time when eating, and to drink at least eight cups of fluid a day. I suggested that water and non-caffeinated drinks were best. I added that processed foods should be avoided, but to eat a small amount of fruit a day. While I was in full flow, I encouraged Ellen to take as much exercise as possible, too.

'I go the gym once a week,' she said, hoping that would be adequate. 'Also I do a fair amount of walking. Isn't that enough?'

'Not bad,' I agreed. 'Really, though, you need a minimum of thirty minutes exercise a day, and three times a week the exercise should make you slightly puffed. As for the stress, exercise will help, and breathing exercises are worth a try. There's a lot of stress in this place, so personally I go running and play a lot of tennis. It all helps.'

I had a leaflet about breathing exercises on my computer, which I printed out. It was an NHS publication on managing your breathing at rest or during exercise. Ellen was happy to take my advice on board and scanned the leaflet with more than a little interest.

Job done, then. And I thought that would be that. However, Ellen developed a more serious expression. Did she have more symptoms? Was another ailment about to be discussed? What was next on the agenda?

'I would like to have a baby.'

'That shouldn't be a problem,' I answered, smiling.

'Apart from those bowel issues, you are fit and healthy. Have you started trying for a baby?'

I assumed I would now have a straightforward doctor/ patient situation where the mother produces the baby and all concerned live happily ever after. That may not have happened with Ricardo and his three lovers, or with Samantha but, even so, I remained optimistic!

Ellen came straight to the point. 'Sorry, I should have said earlier. I'm gay. My partner and I want to start a family but we'll need some help.'

I had no idea that Ellen was gay but I came straight to the point, too. 'Well, this is a "first" for me. We will have a few hurdles to cross, but let's see what can be done.'

As an expert on the birds and the bees I was intrigued to know how Ellen and her partner planned to go about the conception process. Nowadays if you want to be a gay or lesbian parent, there are many options available. A man donates sperm so that a woman can inseminate herself; she can be in a relationship or single; donor insemination can be carried out at home with sperm from a friend or an anonymous donor; and a fertility clinic can use an anonymous donor. Sperm should always be screened to make sure it is free from sexually transmitted infections or genetic disorders, though. In the modern age, lesbian couples who are civil partners at the time of conception, using donor insemination, are treated as the child's legal parents. That also applies to couples who aren't civil partners at the time of conception but conceive through donor insemination at a licensed clinic.

Several years ago, before all of that fell into place, couples like Ellen and Maeve were making it up as they went along, though. So was everyone else, including me.

'I've been with Maeve for a couple of years now. We're letting everyone know that we are a couple. Do you think we should go to a fertility clinic? Do they cater for our needs?'

I paused for a few seconds before answering. I was unsure how the fertility clinic would view two women having a baby together. Normally I had to fill in a multitude of forms before I could refer any couple; I usually had to provide full details about the state of health of the mother and father and also their fertility status. I knew it was usual for a couple to 'try' for three years before they could have any treatment on the NHS.

I had read that sometimes, in the gay community, men offered their sperm for women, so I wondered if they had a sperm donor lined up. I was probing around in the dark, really, looking for the best way forward. 'Would your partner come to see me as well?' I suggested, hoping that three keen minds might be better than two.

'I'm not sure,' Ellen answered thoughtfully. 'She's a bit . . . you know . . .'

'Sensitive?'

'Yes, "sensitive" would be the word. The problem is . . .'

The Turkey Baster

'Go on,' I urged. 'This is all totally confidential.'

'Well, Maeve works in the IT department at the council. They all think that we just share a flat. She's really worried about the reaction she'll get when they find out and whether she'll get a lot of ribbing. She's bisexual, and used to go out with one of the blokes she works with. She hasn't said anything about our relationship to anyone. My friends know about my sexuality, but Maeve hasn't said anything to anyone.'

I paused for a couple of seconds to weigh up the scenario. 'I have to be honest here. I haven't had a case like yours before. If you really are planning to have a baby, though, I can't imagine everything remaining a secret. I reckon it would be a good idea for the three of us to have a chat.'

The following week Ellen appeared with her partner. Maeve had the curliest hair I'd ever seen and the smiliest face ever to light up the surgery. She seemed to have a permanent smile, which meant that a series of laughter lines came and went every few seconds. She wore a denim jacket with jeans – I wasn't sure about denim jackets with jeans, but the dark jacket and light blue faded jeans, sporting a few well-placed 'designer' holes, didn't clash.

'I know Ellen told you about my work situation,' Maeve said as she sat down. 'I "came out", if that's how to describe it, this morning. I told a couple of gossiping types and so everyone will know by now.'

'Why didn't you tell them earlier?' Ellen asked. 'Sorry, doctor, we haven't talked about this much at all. Now seems a good time.'

'I had to be sure of my sexuality,' Maeve said thoughtfully. 'It was complicated, as I used to go out with one of the guys in the team, but the relationship didn't work for me. I gradually realised that I was bisexual, although my strong feelings were for people of the same sex. I feel comfortable in this relationship and it works for me.'

'Did you know that most women are bi-curious? I wrote an article about bisexuality and I won an award,' Ellen beamed, proudly. 'Women become more curious as they get older. A survey was done in America and it involved nearly 500 heterosexual women. Would you believe that sixty per cent were attracted, sexually, to other women? Nearly half of them had kissed a woman with some feeling.'

'That is really fascinating, Ellen; I'd be interested to see your article but we have some forms to fill in,' I said, changing the subject back to the baby issue. 'By the way, which one of you would bear the child?'

Ellen put up her hand like a child in class wanting to go to the toilet. 'That will be me, if possible. Maeve has a higher salary. If we have another child, then it will be her turn, although that is a long way off in the future.'

'Yes, fair enough,' I agreed. 'Mind you, we haven't worked out how we are going to have your first one yet!'

The Turkey Baster

The two women tackled the forms with enthusiasm, but the paperwork wasn't designed for a gay couple. I could see sections to be filled in about the health of the father and providing a sperm sample was out of the question for the parents in this case!

Ellen and Maeve did seem to be a happy, equal, intelligent couple and completely at ease with one another. Personally, I thought that they would make ideal, caring parents.

Maeve joked about the forms and their predicament. 'We'll have to go out looking for men, then. We'll have to persuade them to part with their sperm for a good cause. Maybe one day the authorities will help people like us.'

We filled in the forms, checked them and double checked again. Ellen and Maeve had been totally honest and had given all of their personal details. Would the NHS be able to help?

I heard nothing for three months. There was not a peep from Ellen or Maeve and I wondered whether that could be good news. Perhaps the clinic was trying to find a way to help the couple? As this case was a first for me, I was interested to know how the situation might be resolved, and whether there would be a baby appearing as the end result.

Early on a grey, bleak, Wednesday morning, the rain hammered against the surgery roof. The drops were so large that they exploded into miniature puddles out on the road. I looked out of the window to see Ellen and Maeve weaving their way through the ever-growing pools of water. I checked my list for the day. They didn't have an appointment.

'Dr Leonard is full up this morning,' I heard Doreen say as the couple waited at the reception desk. 'Would it be possible to come back this afternoon? We could fit you in around three o'clock.'

I had a spare few minutes – I was also keen to hear their news – and so I walked through to reception to be greeted by the glum-looking couple.

'Don't worry, Doreen. Mr Clark is always late for his appointments and, for once, I haven't got a long queue of people waiting. I can see them now.'

As Ellen and Maeve came in, I could see from their demeanour that they were both downcast.

'The clinic tried to be helpful,' Ellen said, as tears welled up in her eyes. 'But, in the end, they couldn't help us.'

Maeve took over the explanations. 'Yes, they were really good but they couldn't find a way to start our family. They weren't geared up for our situation and didn't have the budget. We'll have to go private.'

'It's going to cost a lot,' Ellen mumbled gloomily. 'We'll have to have more blood tests and scans to check on the timing of ovulation. Those private clinics charge an awful lot and the hassle would be far too much for us.'

The Turkey Baster

I had to agree that the options were limited. 'Perhaps in the future all of this will be much easier. At the moment, I think you will have to go private. Does that mean, then, that you won't be planning a baby for the time being?'

'We'll have a baby,' Ellen insisted. 'Oh yes, we are in a proper relationship and we would like a child to make our lives complete.'

'We can do it,' Maeve said with a more positive smile, revealing the 'laughter lines' in her face once more. 'There must be a cheaper way. We'll carry out more research and come back to you.'

The rain became even heavier and I could only just hear their parting words. They advanced outside under matching brollies as the howling wind and driving rain hammered away at the surgery. I felt sad that, after all our combined efforts, nothing had been achieved.

'What's up?' Naz asked when the couple had left.

'It's a problem that can't be solved,' I answered as we both filled our cups from the kettle in the tiny kitchen.

'I can guess,' Naz said – she never missed a trick. 'But, on another matter, could you pop into my room for a word? I want to speak to you where we can't be overheard.'

I couldn't help noticing how tidy Naz kept her room. Medical books sat on her desk, forming a carefully constructed pile; a vase of roses – no doubt from a thankful patient – dominated her windowsill; a small oak bookcase displayed a range of medical journals; and her computer glowed from a recent clean.

Just for a change I sat in the patient's chair and waited for Naz to speak.

'It's Dr David,' she informed me, in an official-sounding tone, which was nothing like her normal manner.

'Dr David?'

'Yes, I am very concerned,' she continued. 'Did you know that Kathy, his wife, was ill?'

'No, I didn't,' I admitted, shocked.

Naz had ferreted out all the details. 'No, neither did I, until I was getting petrol the other day and I bumped into his sister. She asked how he was coping at work.'

'He was a bit forgetful last week,' I recalled. 'I did wonder if he had something on his mind. How ill is she? What's wrong with her?'

'She has breast cancer, apparently, and is having all the treatment at the moment.'

'Why hasn't he told us?' Typical stiff upper lip, I supposed.

Naz had been studying her fellow doctor. 'He is coping fine with the patients and their issues, but if you catch him during quiet moments you will see that he is upset.'

'I did notice he was more short-tempered than usual,' I said. 'It was something and nothing. Fiona had a delivery of supplies and the driver had parked too close to the front door. It wasn't a major issue, but he went off at the driver.'

'Would you mind having a word with him to see how he is?' Naz asked. 'You know him much better than I do. Maybe he is coping better than I think. He just needs to be checked out.'

I decided to get straight on the case and knocked at Dr David's door. He'd just seen his last patient for the morning and so the timing was good. The first sight of his face made up my mind for me.

'Don't ask how I found out,' I told him. 'I know about Kathy and it must be really hard for you. How are you coping?'

Dr David adjusted his red silk tie, swept back his silver hair and fiddled nervously with his glasses. 'Well, I didn't want to bother anyone with it but, actually, it's probably best you know about it. Silly really. I thought I was the big, strong man who could cope with any-thing. And when I'm busy I am just about OK, although I do get irritated with patients who come in moaning about nothing.'

I decided not to interrupt.

'You know, it's difficult to control my tongue and not tell them to realise just how lucky they are that they are not genuinely ill,' he said. 'I'm thinking about Kathy now, though, and how her treatment went today.'

'What treatment is she having?'

Dr David went straight into medical mode. 'She hasn't had to have a mastectomy. The whole breast didn't have to come off. It all came as such as shock, though, although it shouldn't have as I've seen it happen plenty of times to patients. She went for her NHS screening mammogram, the one she has every three years, and they found an abnormality.'

'Just in time, then?'

'Yes, it was fortunate,' Dr David continued in his clipped, upper-class tones. 'On the down side, the tumour was malignant. But it hadn't spread to her lymph nodes; they were clear. A classic example of the benefits of screening. They carried out breast-conserving surgery, which was just a lumpectomy, and she's now having radiotherapy. The surgeon said the procedure was usually just as successful as a total mastectomy. They also took away an area of healthy breast tissue around the cancer. Because it's been caught at such an early stage she should be OK. But, of course, it's natural to worry . . .'

'Would you like some time off?' I enquired gently, worried about his reaction.

'Time off? Time off? When did I last have any time off for an illness? I can't have any time off!'

'I think you should,' I said firmly. 'You could give Kathy more support during the day and we could have a locum for a couple of weeks.'

'A locum? A locum?' he boomed. 'My patients

wouldn't know who they were dealing with. That's a daft idea.'

'No, it's not daft,' I insisted. 'Even doctors are sick, or have illness in their families, and I think you would benefit from a break. Remember we are human, like everyone else. And if you are stressed, you are more likely to make a mistake, or have some patient make a complaint about you. And that would only make your stress worse.'

'I can cope,' he blurted out. 'You're just making a fuss . . .'

'Let me go and make us both a cup of tea.'

This was a tactic we all used when Dr David had an explosive moment. We allowed him to calm down, take stock of the situation, and see everything more clearly. Even I was stunned at how well this tactic worked, though, when I returned for round two of our conversation, complete with the tea and a couple of his favourite chocolate biscuits.

'Who would this locum be?' a pensive Dr David asked. 'Could we check out him or her out first? We have built up such a good name that we need the very best doctor. I don't want someone who the patients don't want to see.'

I had an answer ready. 'Do you remember a couple of years ago when Naz went off on maternity leave? We had a Welsh locum – I'm sure he was called Dr Thomas. He was very good. He came from an agency. I'll check my files.'

Doctor's Notes

'Dr Thomas? Dr Thomas?' My distinguished colleague's voice seemed to echo as I strode back to my room to check on the computer.

I returned with a triumphant grin. 'Sorted. He's just finished a stint of maternity cover and can do a couple of weeks from Monday. As this is Thursday, you could tidy up here tomorrow and spend some quality time with Kathy over the next few weeks.'

'It's a deal,' Dr David said, looking relieved and holding out his hand to give me his firmest handshake. My hand took a few seconds to recover. 'And, Rosemary, thank you. I would never have asked for leave, but it probably would be better all round if I have some time off. I've not been sleeping terribly well.'

Later that day, I told Naz all about the developments with Dr David and I could see that she was delighted. In the past she had also used the tactic of leaving Dr David to stew and returning to make him see sense. What a result, we both thought. His work hadn't been too badly affected so far, but we believed we had chosen the correct path to ensure that that did not happen.

A couple of months later, I noticed a familiar name on my list of patients for the day – Ellen! I wondered what lay in store. I was prepared for issues with her bowels, fertility or something completely different.

'Hello, Dr R. How are you?'

'I'm fine, but you're the patient,' I reminded her with

a laugh. 'I saw your name on the list and couldn't help thinking about your previous visits. I asked myself whether it would be bowels or a new condition.'

'I have some surprising news.'

'Oh? Tell me more.'

'Begins with B,' Ellen hinted.

'Bowels,' I guessed, not quite sure where this was leading.

'BABY,' she yelled, hopping up and down inside her mass of baggy, pink clothes. 'What a result. What a result. I'm pregnant!'

'Congratulations,' I laughed out loud, taken totally by surprise. 'I thought you would have given up on that one with all the hassle and expense. Are you sure?'

Ellen was in no doubt. 'My last period was seven weeks ago and I've had a couple of positive pregnancy tests. I had to be totally sure before telling anyone. So, now I am pregnant I have told everyone, including the good Dr Leonard. Could you broadcast the news on radio and everywhere else?'

'I'll see what I can do,' I joked. 'But I can't make any guarantees, so we may just have to tell people by word of mouth. By the way, how much did it cost? Those fertility clinics can cost a small fortune.'

'Guess,' Ellen urged.

'No idea,' I responded. 'Two thousand?'

'Less than that,' Ellen answered. 'It cost a lot less.'

'One thousand five hundred? I honestly have no idea

– I don't know what treatment you had and what the rates were.'

'OK, I'll tell you,' Ellen smirked.

'Go on, then,' I pressed her.

'One pound ninety-five pence.'

'What? I don't believe you.'

Ellen was in her element. 'Yes, the total cost, before expenses, was less than two pounds.'

'Under two quid for state-of-the-art fertility treatment,' I mused. 'Tell me more.'

'Here is the story, then,' she began in a wavering, excited tone. 'We chatted to some gay friends about our situation and we received offers of sperm. Two men came forward and offered to be donors.'

'Is that all legal?' I asked. 'I've had previous experiences of trying to establish the identity of a father.'

'Well, Maeve studied law at university before going into IT, so she's pretty clued up. Both men signed away their rights as a father and Maeve has all the paperwork.'

'Well, I'm not a lawyer,' I admitted. 'Did you say that two men were donors?'

'Yes, the men are two of our close friends. Both provided us with semen samples and we put them in the freezer. The guys are quite similar in appearance – both tall and dark – so we would have been happy with either as the father.'

'I've never heard of anything like this,' I confessed. 'I

assume you had plenty of semen to work with. How could you possibly decide which one to use?'

'This is going to surprise you,' she teased.

'Go on and surprise me. I have absolutely no idea what's coming next.'

Ellen knew that she had me hanging on her every word. Her journalism training ensured that I was totally hooked on her story. 'We thawed the samples and mixed them together.'

'You mixed them together!' I gasped.

'Yes, when they were totally thawed we gave them a really good mix. That meant we had as much sperm as possible and it kept everything vague as to the identity of the father. We stirred and we stirred until the mix was perfect. I had an ovulation kit – oh, I should have included that in the cost – and so I knew when the timing was right.'

'What next?' I asked, intrigued.

'I used a turkey baster.'

'Sorry?'

'Yes, you know those things that suck in the liquid and then pump it out again. I bought it online for £1.95. I loaded the turkey baster with the sperm mixture and we squirted the lot into the top of my vagina. The actual product was called a Graduated Non-stick Turkey Baster.'

I thought to myself that this would make an amazing short story. 'Who did the squirting? Was it Maeve, or a combined effort?'

'To be fair, it was Maeve. We had candles round and a romantic meal with a bottle of wine. The absurd situation meant that we collapsed with the giggles. But it worked – and it was a damn sight cheaper and easier than any fertility clinic.'

I was totally, completely and utterly gobsmacked. It had never occurred to me that a simple kitchen utensil would be used in such a way. Thinking about it, the technique made perfect sense. After all, a turkey baster is just a long-tubed suction device; in Ellen's case, it would have spurted out the sperm mixture high up in her vagina.

As it happened, Ellen had an uncomplicated pregnancy and, with Maeve at her side, Ben came into the world a healthy, eight-pound, little boy. That was ten years ago. Since then I've watched both women turn into the most wonderful, balanced parents. Ellen works part-time and does the lion's share of the day-to-day parenting and school runs. Maeve is also very much a doting, caring parent.

Over the years I've got to know them better and have been able to ask questions that might, initially, have been deemed 'un-PC'.

'How is Ben reacting to having two mummies? Is it a problem at school, or with his friends?'

They have always answered honestly. From the moment they had a son, they were aware that he needed to have male role models in his life. They have made sure that he has close bonds with male members of both of their families. Mercifully, they have been entirely supportive. Ben watches football with his uncles and cousins. They also have many heterosexual friends with children and so he has contact with all of those people. And it genuinely seems that no one bats an eyelid because he has two mummies. Ben says himself that he's one of the lucky ones, having two parents who are still together. Many of his friends at school have never known one of their parents; and, in many cases, the mother and father are separated or divorced. Other children flit between two homes, sometimes at opposite ends of the country.

The two men who could be his father are still friends, but they are not close. Neither of them mentions the fact that they gave the sample, and both Ellen and Maeve say they can't tell who the father is. For them it doesn't matter. Of course, it may matter to Ben when he is a little older and DNA testing may rear its head. But, for now, everyone is happy.

The entire saga has also triggered a change in my attitudes. Though I always try to be open-minded, if I'm honest, I did have some inner doubts about how any child could be brought up in a balanced way by two same-sex parents. But this lovely stable family has dispelled those doubts completely. I am genuinely thrilled for Ellen and Maeve; I am pleased to see Ben developing into a beautiful, happy, normal, well-behaved child; and I am delighted that all the others in his life – the family and friends – have come together for the sake of a lovely little boy.

There is one more lasting effect. It is noticeable on Sunday afternoons when I am preparing chicken, or on Christmas day when the festive bird is benefiting from my finely honed cooking skills. There is no way I can use a turkey baster – EVER AGAIN!

CHAPTER TWELVE

AFFAIRS OF THE HEART

Dr Gareth Llewellyn Thomas was already waiting in reception when I arrived on Monday morning. He looked nothing like a doctor. His haphazard manner belonged more to a laid-back university professor or one of those highly educated types who rule the roost with their persuasive arguments in trendy wine bars. But, behind that 'lived-in' front, there was a highly talented doctor.

'If you remember, we shortened my name to Garth, missing out the "e" to save vital seconds in emergencies,' he quipped as he grabbed my hand and shook it vigorously. At least he didn't crush my fingers in the style of Dr David.

'Welcome back to our practice,' I replied, pointing to Dr David's room. A catch-up was needed before our first appointments of the day.

Garth was about half Dr David's age, tall and dark with a full beard and an athletic build. He played rugby, football, tennis and anything else that involved keeping fit.

'How is the old man?' he asked, looking genuinely concerned. 'It must have been difficult for him, working here with a very sick wife in hospital.'

'It was,' I agreed as Naz emerged and peeked round the door. 'He'll be off for a couple of weeks at least. You'll remember Dr Nazareen Khan? I think you had a brief meeting before her maternity leave a couple of years ago?'

'You can call me Garth if I can call you Naz,' he joked. 'Dr Leonard, may we call you Rose?'

'No!' I exclaimed with a horrified look. 'I do love gardening, but you can't call me after a plant! And whenever I've been called Rose, or Rosie, it's been meant in a kind of derogatory way. I know it's a bit of a mouthful, but if you can manage Rosemary, I'd be grateful.' He laughed out loud. 'How is life on the locum circuit?' I asked. 'You still don't want to settle into a practice?' I was amazed that such a good doctor seemed happy to continue working as a locum, with no job security.

'It suits me really well. I know I could earn more if I was a partner, but I like the freedom to take time off to travel – and I'm not ready for partnership responsibility. Actually, I'm not sure that I ever will be. All that paperwork and administration. I prefer just healing the sick – or, at least, trying to. But it's nice coming back to a friendly practice I know.'

'Are you OK with the computer system?' I checked. 'It's recently been updated. Here's your user name and password – give it time when you log in – it's often a bit slow first thing in the morning, like the previous operator.'

'And like me,' he jested. 'I'll call you if I have any problems with either the patients or the computer!'

I left him to it and went to my room to get ready for my first patient of the day.

'I'm sure this Welsh doctor is all right,' Lizzy whispered as she brought me a coffee, 'but couldn't you get a nice Scottish one instead? I know plenty of nice Scottish doctors.'

'As long as he copes with Dr David's unique band of patients, we can let him off for being Welsh. As it happens, I love their lilting accent.'

'What about the Scottish accent?'

'Can't understand a word of it,' I smiled as she left, pulling a face at me.

Later, as I enjoyed the briefest of lunchtimes, my door reverberated to a series of frantic knocks. I hardly had time to say 'come in' before the door swung open and a flustered Garth strode across to my desk.

'I'd forgotten how busy it was here,' he panted. 'I've seen so many people this morning that my head is swimming. How does Dr David cope?'

'He looks at Mr Hill's ulcers straight away before the old boy has a chance to talk about the way the country is going to rack and ruin,' I ribbed him. 'All OK, otherwise?'

'Yes, I'm just not used to the pace here. I need a coffee.'

'Me, too,' I agreed. 'I know I drink too much of the stuff, but it does help to keep me going. I switch to tea in the afternoon now. Thought I'd better try and practise what I preach . . .'

After the snatched coffees, we headed back to our respective rooms. We waved to Fiona as she dashed around carrying a pile of dressings. I could see that our post-lunch patients had arrived a few minutes early.

'Mrs Hudson should be first for me?' I asked Lizzy.

'Yes, she's in the waiting room. She doesn't look herself. I hardly recognised her.'

'I hope she's all right,' Doreen chipped in. 'She's lost so much weight that I didn't realise who it was.'

I was shocked when Mrs Alice Hudson trudged into my room; this was not the Alice I knew. I guessed that she had lost at least a stone. I recalled that, at one time, she looked slim and attractive. Now she resembled a walking skeleton with a gaunt, haunted look.

I first met Alice when she appeared in the surgery with a broken wrist from a skiing accident. I am a passionate skier and so we had a lot to talk about during that appointment. Like me, she enjoyed a winter break on the slopes with a group of friends. After her hospital treatment, she popped in a couple of times to see how the wrist was healing. That was when I discovered that Alice had borderline osteoporosis. She was of slight build, her mother had a curved spine and, as it can run in families, I arranged for her to have a DEXA scan. This is the best way to check bone density.

I treated her with a bisphosphonate, ensured that she had enough calcium in her diet, and saw her yearly for check-ups. Bisphosphonates are a class of drugs that prevent the loss of bone mass and, in some cases, can even promote the build-up of a little new bone. They are used to treat osteoporosis and similar conditions.

Now, a year after her last check-up, Alice looked in a real state. I knew that she worked as an in-house lawyer for a large publishing company. I recalled that she was divorced, with no children, but had come to terms with that several years ago. So why the long face now?

'You don't look your usual cheerful self. Can I help?'

'I am a bit down in the dumps,' Alice said, staring at the floor. 'In fact, it's more than just being down in the dumps.'

I trotted out a predictable response, because it seemed the right thing to ask. 'Any particular reason why?'

'Oh, it's nothing really . . .'

'It has to be something quite serious,' I stressed. 'You look as if you've lost weight.'

'So you noticed. Yes, I have no appetite and, as you

can see, I'm losing weight. I can't afford to lose much more weight or I might just disappear.'

'Do you have any other symptoms? Tummy ache, change in your bowels, shortness of breath? Weight loss can be a sign of a serious underlying illness.'

'I don't think I'm ill in that way,' she reassured me. 'I'm just a bit upset.'

'Upset enough to lose weight and stop eating?'

She looked at the floor.

I realised I'd never asked her if she'd had a new partner since her divorce.

'Man trouble?' I suggested gently.

'I suppose you could call it that.'

I looked at her expectantly.

'I've been having an affair with a married man for nearly thirty years,' she confided.

'That can't have been easy,' I answered, gesturing for Alice to continue with her story.

'No . . .'

'So, is it over?'

'Yes, but in the most terrible way.'

'Do you want to tell me about it?'

'We met when we were in our late twenties. He had a young family and his wife concentrated on the children. He felt ignored and that was why the affair started. It just carried on and on. He ran a firm of surveyors, which meant that he was always out and about. We used his job as a cover for meeting up.'

'Did you think that he would leave his wife for you?' I asked, feeling sad that this highly intelligent career woman had played second fiddle for so long.

'Yes, I thought he might,' Alice confessed. 'But he never did. I often thought about breaking it off. In fact, I stopped seeing him several times, but could never get him out of my head. I wasn't interested in anyone else. Ronald was five years older than me and had packed an awful lot into his life. You could say he lived life to the full. Unfortunately for me, I just enjoyed a few snatched moments of happiness. Those moments were with Ronald.'

'Were you in love with him?'

'Yes, I suppose I must have been in love with him because I couldn't get him out of my mind. Although I tried to move on with my life on a few occasions, we always drifted back together.'

'How could you keep that going for thirty years?' I asked, intrigued. 'It sounds amazing that no one found out.'

'Well, we were fortunate,' Alice mumbled into her handkerchief. 'There were a few close calls but, despite the risks, I kept plugging away. As I got older I realised that the chances of finding someone suitable were pretty slim and I dreaded losing him. Stupidly, I just let the situation carry on.'

'What is the situation now, Alice? What can I do to help?'

'He's died. Ronald is dead,' she wept.

Her answer caught me off guard. I suppose that I was expecting her to say that he'd broken it off, she'd broken it off, or his wife had found out. She told the story as if Ronald was still alive; I assumed that he lived on in her memory and she just could not accept his passing.

'He's dead? Oh my goodness, I am so sorry,' I blurted out. 'I'm so sorry.'

'Thanks, Rosemary,' she cried and spilled more tears into her handkerchief. 'My problem is that I can't tell anyone I am in mourning. I don't exist as far as his family and friends are concerned. No one knew about the affair and so no one, apart from you, knows how I am feeling right now. I can grieve in private, but not in public.'

I sympathised. 'You are all alone with your memories, and no one will ever know what those memories contain.' I asked her how she found out about Ronald's death.

'It was the worst day of my life,' Alice spluttered through a mist of tears. 'Everything was going well for us, apart from all the secrets. He came round to my house at least once a week when he was "away on business". We were due to have lunch on a Friday afternoon and he didn't show up.'

'I take it that he always turned up for your dates, or at least let you know if he couldn't make it?'

'Yes, that was why his non-appearance was so unusual. In all of our thirty years as a secret couple he had always made it to our meetings. A couple of times he had been half an hour late, but that was about it. I sensed that something was wrong, and I just waited and waited in the wine bar. He failed to show up, so I went home.'

I felt really sorry for Alice. She started to cry; I pushed a box of tissues in her direction, as the soaking handkerchief was beginning to feel the strain.

'Three days later, I still hadn't heard anything from Ronald. I pretended to be a client and called his secretary. I just assumed that he had been held up on an appointment, or one of his meetings had gone on a bit. But I couldn't explain his three days of silence. I thought he'd gone off me, or his wife had found out – something like that.'

As Alice continued her tale of woe, I could see that she was shaking. I tried to imagine how traumatic it would be to lose a loved one and keep everything bottled up inside. She explained that, when his secretary broke the news, her world fell apart.

'I just felt so confused,' Alice said, trying to recover her composure. 'The secretary explained that he had been at a meeting, felt unwell and collapsed. She believed that I was one of his clients on the day and so she told me what happened. I couldn't come to terms with it. I wanted to call him, send a letter or whatever, but I could do nothing. Ronald was dead and I had to mourn inside. I had to mourn alone.'

I encouraged Alice to get it all out of her system,

while I assessed the extent of her depression. 'What happened at the funeral?'

'I couldn't go because, as far as everyone was concerned, I didn't even know Ronald. I didn't even tell any of my friends what was going on.'

'Your best friends had no idea what was happening? You must have been tempted to tell someone.'

Alice gave me a stern look, to show that had been impossible. 'No, I couldn't take the chance. I've found out in life that the only way to keep a secret is to make sure it remains a secret. I wanted to visit his grave, but discovered through the grapevine that he had been cremated. I had no idea what happened to his ashes and there was no way of finding out.'

'You've been through the mill, Alice,' I said, trying to comfort her. 'I suggested counselling for another patient whose mother died while giving birth to her. She never knew her mother, and was brought up by her stepmother. She was mourning the death of someone she never knew, but it helped enormously. Would you consider counselling?'

'I don't know how that would help me,' Alice muttered. 'I'm also angry that I got myself into this situation and ruined so much of my life. I'm finding every day really hard. I'll have to go home now, Rosemary. I'm getting too upset.'

Alice wiped away her tears, stood up and walked wearily, with a stoop, out of the room. I saw her to the door and suggested another appointment in a week's time. I thought that, by then, she might entertain the idea of counselling and I was holding off – just – on the option of anti-depressants.

'Call me at any time,' I urged. 'If I'm busy, leave a message with the receptionists and I'll get back to you. Promise that you'll come back in a week's time?'

'I promise,' Alice agreed, with a dismal expression, as she left the surgery and headed off in the direction of her car.

I sat for a while contemplating Alice's plight. All sorts of conflicting emotions were affecting her state of mind. She was enduring such a sense of loss, mixed with regret. Why hadn't she broken it off all those years ago and tried to find someone else? And there was the shame of it all: being a 'mistress'. How would his wife feel if she ever found out? Those thoughts filled my head as I made a note to ensure Alice made her appointment for a week's time.

I was tidying my cluttered desk after Alice's visit when I heard a familiar knock at the door. The knocking technique, with long spaces in between taps, belonged to Dr David – but what on earth was he doing back at the surgery?

'Come in, Dr David. Aren't you supposed to be at the hospital with Kathy?'

'Yes, yes, but she's home now. She's going back as an

outpatient for chemo. I realised I forgot to tell Dr Thomas about Mr Clarkson's recurring bladder infections and how they make him rather confused.'

'Dr David!' I scolded him. 'You have two weeks off. I'm sure Dr Thomas will be able to cope with Mr Clarkson's bladder infection and whatever other conditions he has.'

Dr David was too conscientious for his own good. 'Yes, but I put him on a course of antibiotics. He is due back this afternoon to see if they are working. I also need to . . .'

'It's all on the computer,' I reminded him. 'Dr Thomas will have everything on the screen in front of him and he's more than capable of dealing with Mr Hill and Mr Clarkson.'

'I see. Well, if he needs any guidance, perhaps he could give me a ring?'

'Absolutely,' I replied as I carefully guided Dr David through my door, out of the main door and towards his car. 'I'm sure he'll be able to cope.'

'I heard that,' Garth said as he poked his head around from our coffee alcove. 'For the record, Mr Hill's ulcers are clearing up and I am confident that I can handle Mr Clarkson's bladder and memory problems!'

I grinned and I set off for my room. 'Remember that Dr David has been a doctor for a long time. He's been seeing some of his patients for more than thirty years. Normally, they refuse to be seen by anyone else.

You should consider yourself honoured to take up the mantle.'

'I am, I am,' Garth answered, disappearing back into his room.

'You'll last the pace,' I reassured him. 'Just to warn you, though, you've still to see Mrs Heath. As a heads up, whatever you do, she'll tell you it won't work and you will be wrong . . .'

A week later, Alice was back. Nothing had changed and she looked as glum as ever.

'This is entirely my fault. I've only got myself to blame. The future just looks so bleak.'

'You can't put the clock back,' I told her. 'We all make mistakes. In retrospect, we've all done things which weren't a good idea. But it's all part of life's rich pattern of gaining experience and wisdom.'

My basic attempt at counselling must have found a way through Alice's tough defences. She agreed to try the professional version. Even more help was needed, though, and so I prescribed anti-depressants.

A few months later, Alice was back in the chair opposite my desk, and I could detect no signs of improvement.

'I'm going skiing next week,' I said with a smile, hoping for an enthusiastic response. 'Back to my favourite place on the French-Swiss border. How about you? What are your skiing plans this season?'

'I'm not going anywhere,' she sighed. 'I just can't

face it. If I had a partner I might consider it. When I travelled to the Alps, I used to keep in touch with Ronald. I looked forward to returning home and spending some time with him. Now I have nothing to look forward to.'

I could tell it was going to take a long, long time for Alice to recover emotionally. It usually takes two years to get back to anywhere near a normal state after a bereavement, but I suspected that Alice's broken mind would take a lot longer to heal.

At the time of writing, six years on, she is under the care of a psychiatrist for her depression and is still on medication. But I'm hopeful that she will recover eventually.

'Where is my stapler?' Dr David grumbled as he carried out an early morning sweep of his desk. 'Has anyone seen my scissors? They were in a red tub with my pens. How can I cut anything out of the newspaper without scissors?'

'Dr Thomas wouldn't deliberately hide your stuff,' Naz muttered. 'Everything will be here somewhere. Have a look in your drawers . . .'

As I poked my head around the door, Naz raised her eyebrows at me. I could tell she was trying to be sympathetic and helpful, but her exasperation was clear to see.

'Everything has been moved around. The only object

I can lay my hands on is my computer. Surely he wouldn't have moved my files about in there?'

'Here is the stapler,' Doreen yelled, as if winning a 'find the stapler' contest. 'Look, I just opened a drawer and found the stapler inside. Is there anything else that you can't find, doctor?'

'I left everything in certain places,' my veteran colleague moaned as he fished through the waste-paper bin in a vain attempt to find his letter opener and favourite coaster.

'The letter opener is here beside your pile of elastic bands and not in the bin,' Naz said, sounding at the end of her tether. 'Dr Thomas just moved stuff to suit his way of working. He was only here for a couple of weeks. I'm sure everything will soon come to light.'

'I'm all right now, I'm all right now, I'm sorry.' Dr David sat down on his chair and peered at his computer screen.

'How is Kathy? Has she finished her treatment? An update is in order. Being diagnosed with breast cancer must have turned her world upside down.'

'Yes, Kathy is home again,' Dr David told us as he began to calm down. 'She's OK. Just very tired, but trying hard not to show it.'

'Please keep us posted and if she's not well in any way, let us know. I'd better go – best not to start the surgery late on a Monday morning.'

'Absolutely. Let's get this show on the road . . .' Dr

Doctor's Notes

David's upper-class voice, sounding like an RAF officer from a Second World War film, petered out as I entered my room and prepared for my first patient, who just happened to be another of the 'affairs of the heart' variety. Again, the situation proved to be fraught with difficulties.

'I'm suffering from stress,' Colin said as soon as he sat down in the chair. I could see sweat beading on his brow and he was constantly clenching his fingers. 'I can't eat or sleep properly and my appetite has gone.' I knew I wouldn't have to carry out too much detective work, because Colin clearly needed to open up his heart. 'I'm getting panic attacks and I'm drinking and smoking far too much. You can add to that sweating, headaches and muscles tightening up. Oh, and I have difficulty concentrating. I am feeling at an all-time low . . .' There was a pause. 'And my wife believes that I'm having an affair.'

That was quite an introduction. Colin was a new patient, having moved from North London, and I knew very little about him. I now realised that he was in a frantic state. He was a small man, probably around five feet six inches, with neatly parted black hair. He looked like he was on his way into work, as he was wearing a navy suit, shirt and tie. His eyes looked red – I was unsure if he'd been crying or whether they were a leftover from a heavy night of booze the evening before.

'Why does she think that?' I enquired as Colin

258

trembled in the chair. 'Why does she think you're having an affair?'

'Someone must have told her,' he mumbled.

'And is it true? Are you having an affair?' From what he said, I couldn't work out what was going on.

There was a pause before Colin continued with his sad tale. 'Yes, I suppose I'd better stop the charade and tell you the truth. It's been going on for a long time. I've managed to lead a double life for a few years, but now everything is getting to me. My wife suspects something. So far I've denied it, but I can't carry on like this. I just can't handle it.'

I watched as Colin entwined his hands nervously, scratched behind both ears, rubbed his chin, fiddled with his nose and coughed several times into a clenched fist. The businessman was only forty years old, but he had a lined face and unsightly bags under his eyes. Drinking, smoking, lack of sleep and stress were all taking their toll.

'Please don't tell anyone,' he pleaded.

'I can't tell anyone because of patient confidentiality,' I explained. 'Everything you tell me will go no further. But I think that you should give me some background to see how I can help you.'

'I run a travel company in Tottenham,' Colin continued. 'We've opened a branch down here, so we've moved home as I need to concentrate on building up this branch. I start work at dawn and finish well after dusk. I tried fighting through the traffic for a few weeks but it was too much. The Tube is just too much hassle, so we now live just around the corner. The business is—'

'What about your affair?' I butted in, as I still knew nothing about his wife, the affair or anything else linked to his stress.

'I've been married for twenty years. We have three kids and a good lifestyle. The stressy part is that I've been keeping this enormous secret and I don't know if I can keep it up any more.' Colin seemed to relax a little as he poured out his problems. 'Four years ago my lover had my child,' he revealed, at the same time glancing at me to check for a reaction. 'I met her in Spain while I was visiting one of our resorts and we just fell for each other instantly. We kept it going when we arrived back in this country. I have no idea why we didn't use contraception. We just fell in love, I suppose, and that was it.'

'I take it that you both decided to have the baby,' I answered, keeping my emotions firmly in place and being careful not to seem judgemental about this disclosure.

'I didn't want to have the child,' Colin conceded. 'However, Fran – that is my lover's name – did not want an abortion. To be fair, an unborn child hardly deserves to suffer because of my stupidity.'

'I can see that,' I said. 'How have you managed to keep this double life going for so long?'

'It hasn't been easy,' Colin reflected. 'We're still

having the affair and I go over to see Fran and our son once or twice a week. She lives in Muswell Hill, so it wasn't difficult when I was in North London.'

'And it's all getting too much for you now?'

'I have to admit that I live over this way for more than business reasons. I thought the further I was away from Fran, the better. I can still see her, and more importantly my son, who I love dearly, but she's not in the local area.'

'Colin, this is getting really complicated,' I said. I was aware that, although I was trying hard not be judgemental, I was probably frowning as I worked everything out. 'It's quite a story.'

'It doesn't end there. The little boy is about to start school. The problem is that someone – and I don't know who – has said something to my wife. She has been questioning me about an affair, although there has been no mention of my child. I'm afraid that whoever is feeding her information will spill the beans about my boy.'

'What about your other children?' I asked. 'Which schools do they attend?'

'I have them all in private schools,' Colin continued. 'My little boy's school would have been three miles from our old house. He's starting to grow up, he'll be asking questions, other people will be asking questions, and it's all getting on top of me. Add to that, I'm smoking forty a day and – as you know – I'm drinking far too much.'

'How much do you drink?'

Colin pursed his lips, glanced out of the window and took a few seconds to answer. 'I would say I drink an average of a bottle of whisky a day and three or four beers.'

'That is a dangerous amount,' I warned him. 'With all your smoking and lack of food you are at risk from so many illnesses that I don't know where to begin.'

As I watched Colin twitch and fidget around in his seat, I could see that he was a man in deep trouble. At just after two o'clock in the afternoon, I could detect a stale alcohol smell; last night's session was probably still seeping through his pores.

'And look at what the cigarettes are doing to my fingers,' he grimaced, staring at the yellow stains.

The fingers were the least of his problems. 'If you could see the state of your lungs, you wouldn't have another cigarette.'

Colin coughed, as if to back up my case, and I could hear his chest rattling with the combination of poisons. If ever there was a man who was being ruined by alcohol and cigarettes, it was Colin. He could have starred in an advert warning people not to drink or smoke.

'So that is my story, doctor. I know there isn't going to be an easy fix but I need to get rid of some of this stress before it does my head in. Am I ill, Dr Leonard?'

'Well, I'm not happy about the amount of drinking and smoking,' I told him firmly. 'That will definitely make you ill. Stress isn't an illness – but it can develop into a serious condition if something isn't done. Stress leads to high blood pressure, for example. Chronic stress can lead to depression, so we have to get you sorted out.'

Colin admitted that he felt better having just talked about his problems. He hadn't been able to confide in anyone. Simply by discussing the issues, he was able to release some of his in-built tension. I gave him a selection of leaflets which described stress in great detail and provided some solutions.

'Have a warm bath,' he laughed. 'Listen to music or take up a hobby! Dr Leonard, none of this is going to help me.'

'There's a lot more to tackling stress in there than that,' I said. 'In your case, you can't do much to prevent stress but you can manage those stressful situations more effectively. You can also reduce the impact of stress on your health. You need to reduce the risks of heart attacks, strokes and other life-threatening conditions.'

'Is it that serious?' Colin muttered as his chest rattled.

'It's that serious,' I confirmed.

Colin immersed himself in the leaflet and discovered that some things could make stress worse as well as damaging his health. He also winced when he read about the safe alcohol limits for men. 'It says here that exercise releases a chemical to make you happier and less stressed. Apparently exercise helps you to take out your frustration and anger in a constructive way.'

'That's all true,' I backed up the statement. 'It's worth

reading everything there and, if you feel the need, I can arrange counselling for you. You clearly can't cope with leading a double life. At some point you are going to have to tell your wife. And I think it's better that you tell her before she finds out for herself.'

'I can't tell her – not yet.'

'Think about it, please, before your health suffers even more. This is not going to help any of your children.'

Colin slouched off, grasping his leaflets, with my advice ringing in his ears. He had the option of coming to see me again, taking my advice, or accepting the offer of counselling. He came to see me the following week.

'You were lucky to get an appointment,' I told him when he opened my door. 'There was a cancellation, so Doreen managed to fit you in. Has something changed since we last spoke?'

'Laura has gone into orbit.'

'Sit down,' I beckoned towards the chair. 'What happened?'

'Laura's best friend told her about the affair. She must have seen me and Fran in a pub somewhere and decided to tell my wife.'

'Yes, but you said last time that your wife already knew about the affair,' I pointed out.

'Well, there has been a development,' Colin mumbled as he stifled a chest cough. 'The so-called friend has now told Laura that I have a child with Fran.'

'Oh, you'd better tell me everything,' I said.

'Laura had suspected all along. There must have been various signs that there was more to it than just an affair. Perhaps she found a present for a young boy. Maybe she discovered a note. I have no idea what she came across. She confronted me last weekend and I felt I had no option. I admitted everything. Bizarre though it might seem, I'm not feeling so stressed any more. Everything is off my chest and I'm not in constant panic mode. It's as if I can see all the problems laid out before me now and can tackle them one by one.'

'Well, that makes sense,' I admitted. 'But is Laura going to forgive you?'

'I don't think she'll ever forgive me. But, on the plus side, it seems she is willing to try and make our marriage work. She's laid the law down . . .' I don't blame her, I thought to myself. It's a wonder she didn't thump him as well, or throw him out of the house. 'She's insisted Fran and I have no contact, except when it comes to dealing with our son. He's called Billy, by the way. Laura is quite open-minded and I have to give her credit for that.'

Quite a woman, I thought to myself. I wondered if she would be coming to the surgery for help and support.

Although this was not the expected outcome, I could tell that a huge weight had been lifted from Colin's shoulders.

'I will never stray again,' Colin vowed. 'I have had to endure the worst roasting of my life. Laura really tore into me. I never want to go through that again. Of course,

I deserved every bit of the roasting. And I suspect there will be more to come.'

'Well, it certainly helps that it's all out in the open. But it's not going to be easy for you. We still need to work on your stress, and the booze, the fags . . .'

'Yes, and the worst day of my life is still to come,' he moaned. 'I need to get through it. I will get through it.'

'What will be the worst day?'

'The two women in my life and my love child will all be in the one room,' he gulped. 'After my rollicking, Laura said that we must all meet up, be totally open and honest, and look for a way forward. I know that Laura is furious with me, but she doesn't want to wreck our family. I will be trying to make it up to her for the rest of my life.'

I thought privately that that was a minor punishment for what he had done.

'But I have started reading all the advice. I've started cycling and I'm trying to cut down on the smoking and drinking.'

'Anything else?' I asked, hoping that some of the other anti-stress measures would be considered.

'I had a hot bath and I listened to some music,' Colin jested. 'Seriously, your other suggestions are working for me. If our meeting backfires, I'll be back to see you next week.'

I did see him again, a few weeks later. He was still looking haggard, but better than before.

'Things aren't exactly easy at home. There's an atmosphere. But somehow I can cope with that better than the lies and the deceit. Tell me, Dr R, do you see many people who get their lives into such a mess?'

'Yes, Colin, I do,' I admitted, quite truthfully, knowing full well that as long as I was a GP, I would continue to see hurt and angst from complicated relationships. 'Some mistakes have more consequences than others, of course, and hurt more. But, you know, it's human nature. None of us is perfect. But everyone can learn from their mistakes. You know that phrase, "older and wiser"?' Colin knew what was coming. 'It's so true.'

CHAPTER THIRTEEN

HELPING OUR HEROES

The bright autumn sunshine streaked across the South London sky and a batch of grey clouds light-ened up for a few seconds as the sun forced its way through. Down below, I had enjoyed my journey to the surgery and I walked inside, feeling really good about our reputation. It had taken a long time to build up, through sound medical practice and some cunning detective work, but I really felt we were now on solid ground.

I had to close the roof blinds in my room to see the computer screen. It informed me that the first person on my list that morning was a man called Gavin. He'd registered at the surgery a few years before, but we had no details about him and, as far as I could tell, he'd never actually been into the surgery to see any of us. With young and middle-aged men, that wasn't so unusual. They were usually fit and well but, when they did need medical help, I knew that they often saw doctors either privately in the city, or in one of the many walk-in centres in London.

'Hello, what can I do for you?' I asked, as a middle-aged, nervous man walked in. I could see he walked with a slight limp.

'I've come for some advice, really. I haven't been to see a doctor for years and it took a long time to pluck up the courage, but here I am. I've been in limbo for a while, not doing anything about anything, and my wife made me come to see you.' He looked down at his leg, and I waited to hear what he had to say. 'I was shot while serving in Northern Ireland years ago. I have an artificial lower right leg, and so I gave up driving. I should have taken advice and started driving again, but I didn't.'

'Could I have a look?'

'Here it is,' Gavin showed me, rolling up his trouser leg. 'It's never been comfortable, really, and I've never got my head around using my left foot to drive an automatic car. So, here I am, wanting to drive again and deciding that I should do something about it. I thought I ought to ask you first, though – would there be any problems medically if I started driving again?'

'As long as you don't have other medical problems, then no. If we're only talking about your legs, then it's just a question of getting a car adapted. Have you looked into that?'

A smile beamed across his face. 'Are you sure?'

'I have several disabled patients who drive very safely,' I reassured him, 'but if you've not driven for a while then it would be a good idea to take your time over some lessons, and learn to handle a car with different controls.'

'I've read something about changing the pedals,' he recalled. 'I believe that an extension can be fitted from the accelerator pedal to go on the other side of the brake. I think that's how it works – but I'm not sure that would work for me.'

'Yes,' I agreed. 'And, though I'm no expert on it, I believe if you're not happy with that they can fit controls to use with your hands.'

That was something they don't teach you in medical school, I thought to myself: adapting cars for disabled people.

Gavin's face lit up. 'It would be too difficult to move my left foot over to do the job of a right foot. But I would love to take the family out for the day, and this would give me so much more freedom. I have been lazy, though, and I haven't looked into it. With my war pension and everything, I've been told that I qualify for motability allowances. I need to get cracking on this.'

'Yes, you do need to find out more,' I said. 'I've got one patient similar to you who has adapted their own car, but I think you may even be able to lease an adapted vehicle. It sounds as if it would make an enormous difference to your life. Go for it!'

Doctor's Notes

'I'm on the case.' Gavin jumped up, forgetting his stability problems for a moment and almost keeling over. 'Doctor Leonard, this could change my life. I'll be back with an update.'

Gavin headed off from the surgery with boyish enthusiasm. I peeked out of the window to see a woman, I presumed to be his wife, at the wheel of a people carrier. I could make out two or three children in the back. How wonderful if Gavin could take the controls and transport his family to the seaside . . .

The next appointment on my list was one I was really looking forward to and it promised to be the highlight of my day.

Iain was a pilot who had served in the Battle of Britain and North Africa at the controls of his Hawker Hurricane. He joined the RAF as a real rookie. He said the senior pilots taught them not how to fly, but how to fight.

Iain first flew his Hurricane in the Battle of Britain in 1940, defending Britain's skies against the Nazi war machine. During previous appointments to keep a check on his high blood pressure, Iain had said little about the war. Now with Armistice Day approaching, he decided to open up.

'We were vastly outnumbered by a ruthless enemy but we sent them packing,' Iain told me, with a triumphant look on his face. 'The Luftwaffe came at us with two and a half thousand planes when the Battle of Britain started.

Helping our Heroes

We only had a few hundred serviceable fighter aircraft. Did you know that? Those air battles were horrible – planes were blowing up all over the sky.'

'I wasn't sure of the exact figures but I knew that the RAF fought against all the odds,' I replied.

'Yes, those Nazis thought they could wipe us out in four days, and they tried their darndest. They should have tried to finish off our airfields and radar installations, but they didn't. They went for cities, instead, in an effort to destroy morale. Can you imagine the British people surrendering?'

'That would never happen,' I agreed. 'If anything, the threat from an enemy makes us more determined to fight for our values. It's always been that way.'

'The Germans' blunder gave us time to regroup. They underestimated the importance of radar which told us when their planes were coming. And then we had a few aces up our sleeves – Spitfires and Hurricanes.'

'What were they like to fly?' I asked, totally hooked on the veteran's story, and blowing all hope of running my surgery on time. 'How did the Hurricane compare to the Spitfire?'

'Well, the Spitfire handled like a dream. She handled like the finest lady I have ever known, and I've known some fine ladies. The aircraft was so easy to handle, and it was so fast and so powerful. I spent most of my time in a Hurricane, though, and that was more of a workhorse. She wasn't so fast and didn't climb so well. However, she took a lot of flak and was really robust and stable. And we could out-turn the German Me109. That always shocked the German pilots.'

Talking to Iain was like receiving a really interesting history lesson. 'But you must have been afraid. I can't imagine dicing with death every day. I've seen old films of battles in the air and it all looks pretty grim.'

'Well, if you were scared, you couldn't show it or admit it. Of course, there were terrifying moments. When you know that you are in the sights of an Me109, your life races past in your mind. And we were all so young. But we couldn't let our mates know that we were afraid to die. Mind you, as our life expectancy was only four weeks, a large number of pilots didn't survive the war anyway.'

Iain's eyes misted over as the memories flooded back. 'My luck ran out during a savage dogfight. The plane was badly shot up and I took a few hits myself. I managed to coax the aircraft home, but I took a lot of punishment. The surgeons did an amazing job because I almost bled to death. Look, I still have the bullet holes.'

'Yes, you've shown me those before,' I reminded Iain as he opened his shirt to reveal a selection of scars. He was fortunate that the shrapnel had missed vital organs. I was amazed that he was still alive, enjoying life in his eighties and packing a lot into every day.

'Iain, your story reminds us of how much this country owes to the sailors, soldiers and air crews who saved us from invasion,' I said, overcome with admiration for my patient and his fellow pilots. 'We mustn't forget the young men from all sides who were sent into battle. It's bizarre that old enemies are now meeting up, discussing the dogfights and enjoying drinks together. I can cure a few ailments here, but time is also a great healer.'

'I'm still trying to do my bit,' he continued. 'I've been working with an organisation that helps limbless ex-servicemen and women. We're trying to make life more comfortable for troops who've lost their arms or legs. There are so many casualties returning from Afghanistan, you know. We also try to help dependants and widows.'

Iain couldn't be stopped when he was in full flow, and I actually encouraged him. 'What do you do to help?'

'We give advice on provision of artificial limbs and nursing care,' Iain continued. 'Then there is counselling, disabled sport, advice on war pensions, transport for disabled people and a whole lot more. We've got Armistice Day coming up, too, and that's a huge occasion among the veterans around here.'

'I'd better check your blood pressure,' I said, looking up at the clock. 'I assume that's really why you came to see me!'

'Yes, I know I should have it checked more often at my age. You did tell me last time that high blood pressure increases the risk of a heart attack or a stroke.'

'Yes that's right. I check blood pressure all the time, especially with so many senior citizens as patients. It's known as the silent killer, not that you are in any danger at this precise moment!'

'Do a lot of people my age have high blood pressure then?' Iain asked, switching his interest from air battles to medical matters.

'In England, around thirty per cent of people of all ages have high blood pressure but a large number don't know it. You should have your blood pressure checked often, but all adults should have it checked at least every five years.'

Iain enjoyed hearing details and facts and figures. 'What is blood pressure, anyway?'

'It is the pressure of blood pressing against the cells of your arteries as it is pumped through the body. Your heart and arteries feel the strain if the pressure is too high. "Systolic pressure" is the pressure of the blood when your heart beats. "Diastolic pressure" is the pressure of the blood when your heart rests in between beats. Your blood pressure is 140 over ninety,' I said as I carried out the test. 'So your systolic pressure is 140, and your diastolic pressure is ninety. The numbers represent millimetres of mercury. It would be great to bring that down from 140 to around 130.'

'How do I bring my blood pressure down?'

'Keep taking your medication,' I advised. 'Remember to cut down on your salt intake and eat plenty of fresh fruit and vegetables. Keep eating a low-fat diet and make sure it includes lots of fibre. You don't drink or smoke, so that's good, and you don't have too much caffeine. Oh, and keep doing plenty of exercise.'

'Keeping to that list will kill me,' Iain joked as he stood up and made his way out of the surgery.

A few weeks later another hero of mine appeared in the surgery; again he had survived brutal wartime battles, this time in a Spitfire. Jack lost his legs during the war. He didn't like to talk about the dogfights and I was reluctant to press him for details, or mention Iain's battles in the skies.

Jack has been a patient for my entire career as a GP, and was in his mid-sixties when I first met him. He always looked dapper and trim, and around a decade younger than his actual age. During our first meeting, I noticed that he had an odd gait as he came into my room. He had two prosthetic legs below the knee. He was shot down during a dogfight and his legs were blown away.

Now, as he hobbled into my room more than twenty years later, I was filled with admiration and respect for this veteran of the skies. Like Iain, he was also helping our modern-day heroes by raising money to help limbless ex-servicemen and women.

I could tell that Jack was in pain, as he winced while attempting to stride into the room. His face contorted for a few seconds as he moved awkwardly towards the patient's chair. Jack had had his right hip replaced and I hoped he wasn't overdoing things. Both hips had shown signs of advanced arthritis; the right hip gave him more trouble than any other part of his body.

'Are you taking your painkillers, and how are the exercises going?' I asked as Jack sat down.

'Well, I take the painkillers when I really have to. I'm doing the exercises all the time. If they hurt too much, then I stop. I'm getting out and about as much as possible, which means staying as fit as I can.'

I gave Jack a full check-up and, despite his age, I could see that he was in remarkably good condition. I sent him on his way with a promise from him that he'd come back for another check-up soon.

The next day, as I snatched a few minutes between appointments, Fiona came bursting into my room. Her hair was not styled in its usual manner and her blue eyes failed to dazzle; those eyes, normally sparking, were filled with sadness.

'Fiona, what on earth is the matter? Is everything OK with your family? Has your dog recovered from her operation?'

'Oh yes, everything is OK there,' she said, deep in thought about something else. 'I've just been to the bank and it really made me think. Something has really got to me.'

'Bad service again?' I suggested. 'I know I had to wait in a long queue the other day. I gave up and tried the cashpoint, but it was out of order so it was a complete waste of time.'

'No, no, nothing like that,' she mumbled, still with a sad expression. 'The customer in front of me was a young lad in a wheelchair without any legs and only one arm, and two of the fingers on that were missing. Well, he just had short stumps. He was carrying bank cards in a small bag round his neck and he looked so awkward using just his remaining fingers to get them out. He was withdrawing twenty pounds, and I just felt so humble and helpless standing there. I overheard him telling the cashier he'd been blown up in Afghanistan.'

I nodded, 'There are quite a few service people coming back from the front line with awful injuries. The older veterans are actually raising money to help them.'

The sight of the young lad had really affected Fiona. 'I just thought to myself: I had all my limbs, present and correct, and everything I needed to carry out the transaction at the counter. This young lad had obviously decided to remain independent and he was performing miracles, just by withdrawing his cash.'

I nodded in agreement. 'I was reminded of the horrors of war when a veteran pilot came in to the surgery. This young man you saw – is he from around here?'

'He was from a local regiment,' Fiona confirmed. 'I overheard his conversation with the cashier. Anyone could see he was a soldier because he had his uniform on and a crest of arms on his wheelchair or buggy thing. He was no more than twenty years old, for sure.'

I was now becoming concerned for the brave young soldier. 'What had happened to him?'

'Well, he was saying to the cashier that he was blown up by one of those roadside bombs. His two mates were killed and he wasn't expected to survive. I heard him say that, when he realised he was still alive but with no limbs, he vowed to carry on for his mates. I put five pounds in his tin – he was raising money for a charity to help limbless servicemen and women,' Fiona added as her determined look returned.

'Which charity?'

'I'm not sure,' Fiona replied, scratching her chin. 'It said something about raising money for soldiers who were injured in Afghanistan. I did ask him about it when he'd finished at the counter. He said he was all sorted out with his equipment, but more money was needed to make life comfortable for some of his friends. I also bought a poppy, because he was handing those out as well. Why do you ask?'

'Well, all these veterans are doing exactly the same thing,' I explained. 'I've been hearing about charities, similar to the one you mentioned. How amazing that the young lad is raising money for limbless ex-service people, too. The veterans and the young soldier were all fighting for our country, many years apart, and they're both now involved in the same projects. Put five pounds in for me if you see your soldier friend again.'

'My family lost loved ones in both World Wars, so I'd be keen to help out,' Fiona told me.

That summed up Fiona perfectly. Once she latched on to a subject she gave it 100 per cent. I knew that she would track down the soldier in the wheelchair. She headed off in the direction of her treatment room and I carried on with my surgery.

Later that week, Fiona appeared in my room, overflowing with enthusiasm and carrying a pile of leaflets. She was in such a hurry that some of the leaflets toppled from the pile and floated down to the floor.

'I have all the info,' she spluttered. 'All the gen is here. Look, here are all the details about the parade through Dulwich on Remembrance Sunday. I've never been to that service before. I'll certainly be going along this time. There's a school band and cadets from the Army, RAF and Royal Navy. I saw the young soldier in the wheelchair again and he gave me all the bumf.'

'Let's have a look,' I said, picking up one of the leaflets from the floor. 'Yes, the Combined Cadet Force will be marching to Christ's Chapel at Dulwich College. There are lots of other events happening, so it should be quite a spectacle. There's the traditional two-minute silence and another parade afterwards. My sons must know something about it – they aren't in the school's Combined Cadet Force, but they sing in the chapel choir. If they are involved, I'll pop along, too.'

'See you there,' Dr David poked his head around the door. 'You lot have been mustering up plenty of enthusiasm for Sunday. I was just a small child during the war but I remember seeing all of the soldiers, sailors and air crews on duty around London. Vague memories, mind you, but they're still there.'

When I got home, I found out that my sons did, indeed, know about the Remembrance Day March in Dulwich. They recalled that a lot of 'standing around doing nothing' was involved, and apparently someone always faints. One fateful year some girls from one of the local schools had been to a party the night before, had a late alcoholic night, and so were not on best form the following morning. Several of them had keeled over 'like dominoes'. The challenge for the other youngsters was not to giggle. The challenge for the staff was to try to stop the whole row of girls going down. Now, apparently, there was some sort of sweepstake about how many were going to faint each year from each school. Not too respectful to the dead, I thought, but at least they were attending.

Remembrance Sunday arrived and I wore a black coat. I pinned my poppy on the left side – some people wear it on the right but at the BBC everyone pins it on the left, so I followed suit. I watched the march to Christ's Chapel and was pleasantly surprised to see such a large turnout. There were soldiers, sailors, aviators, cadets and spectators of all ages lining the streets. I smiled as I saw my boys parading along the road with their school friends.

Not a sound could be heard during the two-minute silence and, more importantly, I thought with my medical hat on, no one appeared to have fainted. During the Last Post, the bugler, a young musician from one of the schools, played without the slightest interruption. He'd clearly been practising.

All around the college, nothing moved. As the wreaths were laid at Christ's Chapel, I spotted a familiar, stooping figure at the back of the gathering. Iain was wearing an old-style, RAF, blue-grey uniform, with his wings, medals and other insignia denoting the presence of a hero. I assumed that Jack would be here, too, somewhere, among the hundreds of people paying their respects.

It was hard to remember seeing so many souls in Dulwich at the same time. I even caught sight of Dr David, with his dark suit and black tie, soaking up the atmosphere, along with his wife. I was delighted to see that Kathy looked remarkably well, despite all her health problems. I could sense that they felt privileged to be standing there, paying their own tributes. I caught a glimpse of Fiona and her family, and Lizzy towered above the onlookers at the side of the chapel. It was quite a turnout from the surgery; I suspected that Fiona hadn't just been talking to me about the injured soldier.

As the ceremony drew to a close, I inched my way over in Iain's direction. He was alone at the service and I could see that he was alone with his thoughts as well. Tears filled his eyes as he remembered the gruelling wartime battles and the deeply felt loss of his comrades. I thought to myself that wartime pilots must be few and far between; there weren't many 'Iains' in the lines of spectators. We were indebted to the few in the Battle of Britain who were left.

Iain was also paying tribute to troops on the ground, as he quietly repeated the words of some wartime poems, written by troops in the trenches. He even knew the words to a poem by a German soldier, and I thought that was important; victims from all sides had to be remembered. I walked over and stood beside him.

'Hello, doctor,' a voice behind me said. 'What a poignant service that was. I see your friend there, reading out some poetry. I wrote a short poem for today. I've been reading up about the First World War and some words just came to me.'

I was delighted to see Gavin. Before I had the chance to ask him about his car issues, he prepared to launch into verse.

'What's it called?' Iain and I asked at once, as Gavin opened up his notebook.

'It's called "The Gun and the Flower". It speaks for itself, really.'

'Off you go, then, lad, let's hear it,' Iain urged as Gavin fumbled to find the right page. I could see there were lines of verse throughout the book, all in his handwriting.

Gavin held his book, like a vicar reading out a hymn during a church service. 'Here it is, then, "The Gun and the Flower".'

Iain stood to attention as he listened; I had no idea what to expect. Gavin twitched nervously and the grey sky turned black as threatening clouds rolled in. Leaves swirled all around as the bare trees prepared for winter, while the veterans chatted to their families about lost comrades.

> *I see young men; they yell, they charge*
> *Onwards into battle*
> *Machine guns speak; they shout aloud*
> *They talk with a deadly rattle*
>
> *The enemy, just over the hill*
> *The enemy, cutting us down*
> *The fallen, screaming at my feet*
> *The fallen are all around*
>
> *And yet I see a flash of green*
> *A flower opens up its eyes*
> *The flower weeps; the machine gun speaks*
> *Then, like my friends, it dies.*

Doctor's Notes

I was stunned, and felt quite emotional. 'Gavin, that was wonderful,' I said. 'I'm lost for words.'

'I hadn't expected that,' Iain told him. 'It must have been absolute hell in the trenches during the First World War. My father fought in that war and, from what he told me, it was exactly like that. The men were just cut down as they climbed out of the trenches. If they turned back, they were shot for cowardice. The worst thing was the fate of the Scottish pipers. They were unarmed and led the troops into battle. Lines of them were simply massacred. Although I fought in the Second World War, many of my thoughts are with those who served between 1914 and 1918.'

There was nothing else to be said about the poem or the centuries of wars. Gavin seemed to have summed up the futility of it all, with even the flower of hope perishing in the carnage. It was time to move on and talk about his transport issues.

'That's my car over there,' Gavin announced with more than a little pride. 'I couldn't get on with the change of pedals, but I qualified for a car with hand controls. Look at that!'

I was delighted to see a brand new Ford, sunroof open despite the November chill, parked halfway along the street. I knew that the vehicle was going to a deserving cause and felt quite pleased with myself for what I had done to help. This time, there was no sign of the wife and kids. I presumed that they had deliberately allowed Gavin to pay his respects alone.

286

Our afternoon was far from over.

'Hello, my name is Bob. Are you Dr Leonard? You look like that doctor on the telly.'

'Yes, that's me,' I answered as Bob showed off his medals to a crowd of admiring onlookers. 'I assume that you come here every year?'

'Yes I do, and I hope to see many more parades as long as my health holds out. I seem to be the only veteran who is still in one piece.'

'I can tell,' I said, as Bob saluted a group of fellow comrades.

'I am registered at your practice, but I haven't been to see a doctor for years. I'm fine apart from my hearing. It was damaged by an explosion on the ship I was serving on.'

'Oh? What happened?'

'Well, it all kicked off in the Med in 1944. I was serving on a minesweeper and we were completing a sweep when a mine exploded on board. There were many casualties. I was only a short distance away and my ear drums took the full force. I'm lip reading as you talk!'

'Come to see me any time,' I told my elderly new patient. 'I'll give you a proper check-up and I can refer you to the audiology clinic to check that you have the best, up-to-date hearing aid.'

Next there was a completely unexpected development.

'Hello, are you Dr Leonard? I've been looking for

you. You could be just what the doctor ordered, as they say.'

The voice came from a crowd of people and I couldn't be sure who had mentioned my name. I peered through the mass of black suits and poppies, but still couldn't work out who was talking to me. Then I saw a soldier's uniform, a smiling face, a body with no legs, one arm and a juddering wheelchair.

'I hear that you're interested in saving Private Ryan and some of his mates?' said the young man in the chair. 'Well, I'm Ryan, as you've probably guessed. Fiona over there told me that you were interested in helping us lot when we come back in bits from Afghanistan. Well, I came back in bits and I'm on something of a crusade.'

I could see that Ryan's arms and legs had been blown away and he was operating the wheelchair with his one remaining hand on an electric control. His stumps attached to crutches, allowing him to make contact with the ground. I waved to Fiona as she left the service and welcomed Ryan into our impromptu gathering. I put my hand on his shoulder as a greeting, and Iain and Gavin did the same.

'Fiona said she saw you at the bank,' I said, marvelling at the mobility of Ryan's wheelchair. He had the operation down to a fine art, manoeuvring backwards and forwards, turning right and left or coming to an abrupt halt.

'Yes, with a little persuasion she agreed to help

our campaign,' Ryan grinned. 'It's just a case of raising awareness about the problems facing people like me and finding cash for some extra comforts and activities. We do get help, but I'm pushing for extra counselling, more spending money, family holidays, better pensions and a whole lot more.'

Ryan gestured towards the basket on his wheelchair where a photo album had pride of place. I opened it and saw limbless veterans skiing, skydiving, sailing and climbing mountains. I could tell at once what a difference all this made; the veterans were having the time of their lives, using whatever limbs and energy they had to the maximum. I put five pounds in Ryan's tin and filled my pockets with leaflets.

'That's your second fiver,' Ryan pointed out, handing the note back to me. 'Fiona put in five pounds for you the other day.'

'Money well spent!' I declared, stuffing the note back into the tin. 'It would only buy me a couple of coffees, so I'll just do without the coffees.'

Iain looked enviously at Ryan's tin and, fortunately, I had enough money in my purse to add to his collection. 'Here you are, Iain. I think you both deserve a fiver.'

'You've just saved Private Ryan and a veteran airman,' the soldier in the wheelchair laughed. 'If you could hand out those leaflets and spread the word, you might see me climbing a mountain soon. I might need a wheelchair ramp, but hey . . .'

Doctor's Notes

As I smiled and prepared to leave, I was aware that Ryan was gesturing towards the college building with his one remaining arm.

'There is one person that we haven't mentioned today. I saw wreaths for him but he is worth bringing up in our conversation. In fact, he's worth a big mention; I didn't know him but I've been told a lot about him.'

'Who are you talking about?' I asked, puzzled.

'I'm talking about an ex-pupil of that college over there. Lieutenant Mark Evison, First Battalion Welsh Guards, officer commanding Seventh Platoon. Everyone talks about him all the time.'

'I saw his obituary in the newspaper,' I told our small, respectful gathering. 'Why is Mark remembered with such affection?'

'I've heard that he was a top bloke,' Ryan said, softly. 'The Commander of the Welsh Guards said he was the best platoon commander in the regiment. The Commander was actually killed in action as well, soon afterwards, but he sent Mark's mum a letter all about her son.'

We all waited while Ryan regained his composure and continued his story.

'Mark was trying to find members of his platoon who hadn't made it to safety during a patrol in Helmand Province. He was shot in the shoulder and lost an awful lot of blood. He was brought back to this country, but died in hospital with his family at his bedside.'

Helping our Heroes

We all turned to look at the college's war memorial, which was now bedecked with wreaths.

'Here you are,' Ryan thrust a newspaper cutting into my hand. 'I'm from a different regiment, but I live in Dulwich and we all pay our respects to Mark.'

I read the newspaper cutting, which described how Mark had a gift for music. He attended Dulwich College Prep School, and then Dulwich College itself. He won a music scholarship in cello and piano to Charterhouse School. After that he went on to Oxford and Sandhurst.

'Oh and don't forget that Mark was one of the fittest men in the Army,' Ryan shouted out. 'At the age of seventeen he ran the London Marathon in three hours fourteen minutes. I didn't even know the bloke, but he was a fine leader of men.'

'What a character,' I almost gasped as I read more of the article. 'It says here that he managed a sheep farm in Australia and attempted to become the youngest person to walk to the South Pole.'

The article reported that Mark's mother, Margaret, had established the Mark Evison Foundation. It gives financial support to young people who have a goal they want to achieve, which will contribute to their own personal, physical and mental development.

I agreed to do what I could to help the veterans and their causes. Ryan, Iain, Jack, Gavin and Bob had climbed so many mountains in their lives already; I was more than happy to help our heroes with the monumental challenges that lay ahead.

It was business as usual at the surgery the next day. With winter fast approaching, the season of coughs and colds was starting, and as I walked in, I could hear sneezes and snuffles coming from the packed waiting room. My head was still filled with the experiences of those brave servicemen I'd met the day before. All of their stories made me so proud to be an important part of the community; knowing what they had been through made life in South London seem like a picnic!

I looked out of my window to see Dr David huffing and puffing as he tried to fit his enormous Jaguar into a small parking space. Doreen and Lizzy were already in position manning the telephones, and I could hear Fiona and Naz having a medical chat outside the treatment room.

I scanned my list for the day and assessed the probable conditions and treatments. Oh, and I also made a note of a few possible investigations – Detective Leonard at your service!

Doctor, Doctor

DR ROSEMARY LEONARD

Incredible True Tales from a GP's Survery

'Hello, this is the emergency services. Do you require fire, police or ambulance?' asked the female switchboard operator with brisk professionalism.

I thought fast. 'I actually need all three,' I answered.

It's not every day that a home visit turns out to be an eco-protestor with appendicitis stuck up a tree. But as *BBC Breakfast*'s Dr Rosemary Leonard shares in this book, it's all part of a day's work for a South London GP. From an octogenarian nymphomaniac to a teenager in labour with a baby she didn't know about, when Dr Rosemary opens her surgery door she doesn't know who's going to walk in . . .

'A riveting read' *Daily Express*

'She has a breezy, confident style that makes this an entertaining glimpse into the sharp end of medicine' *The Lady*

'Funny, heartwarming . . . and you can skip the gory bits' *Yours*